FIFTY SHADES OF SEXUAL FANTASY

BY DARBY JONES

The primary aim for this book is to share knowledge and to entertain. It is completely free from copyright restrictions.

If you purchased this book: Thank you for supporting my work! Your purchase motivates me to continue to produce new material. Every sale is important to me, both financially and personally. Please feel free to share this book with all of your friends.

If you did not buy this book: I hope that you enjoyed reading this book. I understand that limited distribution networks mean that this book is not available for sale in many parts of the world or even to those without credit cards. I also understand that for many people, filesharing networks are the only way to access ebooks like this. If you enjoyed this book then please help spread the word by voting it up and leaving positive reviews on the tracker site where you found it. Please support private trackers with donations whenever possible.

TABLE OF CONTENTS

INTRODUCTION

Thanks to books like The Secret Garden and Fifty Shades of Grey, sexual fantasy is becoming ever more mainstream. This book has been written to help you create your own delicious recipes for indulgent sexual pleasure. In these pages you will discover fifty exquisite, sensuous fantasies that will transform your sex life into a series of exotic adventures that would have made even Casanova and Madame de Pompadour green with envy. Online shopping means that there are now more toys, games and sexy outfits available than ever before. This book is an intimate guide on how to put all these products to their best possible use. All of the suggestions here are tried and tested and guaranteed to add much more than a spark to your sex life. They will bring a bang to your bedroom that you will not believe.

A rich and fulfilling sex life is something that is available to everybody regardless of class or culture. In a society where everything becomes more expensive by the day, sex is one of the few pleasures that we can all enjoy at little or no cost. The only requirement is vivid and fertile imagination. Sex, just like love and music or poetry and painting can be a source of endless delight. It is a far more memorable experience than any blockbuster movie, video game or expensive holiday. Despite all our technological advances, sex is still the most rewarding experience known to man. It is even said that some women enjoy it too!

The Importance of Play

At its most basic level, imaginative sex is simply a form of play. But just because it is play does not mean it is unworthy of attention. Everything is better when it is naturally fun. If you think that all play is silly, or a waste of time, you will probably not understand imaginative sex, or, for that matter be very good at it. Play can be very beneficial if the proper perspective is taken. It is after all the most effective way of

1

learning. Play can also be taken very seriously. Once play moves into the realms of sport and games, things are taken much more seriously. Look for example at how people play chess. Or football or any other form of organised sport for that matter. In reality they are only forms of play. Have you ever taken part in a sport which you absolutely love? It is so much more than just physical exercise because you enjoy it so much. So many things are better when they are done having fun. The best work is fun. The best work feels more like play, because it gets you into a flow state. Play in any situation, can stimulate the mind, increase energy and and provide a healthy outlet for stress and tension. In a love context, it is a catharsis for bottled emotions and suppressed desires.

Although our sensationalist modern media emphasises only the physical aspects which it can commercialise, sex is in fact primarily centred in the brain. If the brain is so important in sexual matters, then obviously our imaginations should be able to enhance our sexual lives. Imaginative sex is delightful, exciting and, very pleasurable. Many medical professionals support the therapeutic value of imaginative sex. Common sense alone tells us that it has very valuable potential. Drama can have a profoundly cathartic effect, release emotion, energy and self-understanding. Imaginative sex can be a sane and healthy way to express one's darker desires. We all possess elements of both dominance and submissiveness, though in varying ratios. In every human being there are certain sadistic elements and certain masochistic elements. These darker aspects are seen as natural, part of our evolutionary past. They cannot be denied, ignored, repressed or forgotten. The key is for each person to find a way to express these feelings in a way that is sane and healthy. Entering into the fantasy world of another human being can be a very stimulating and exciting experience. We do not know another person, really, until we know their fantasies. The intimacy that develops when two people share their innermost fantasies can solidify their relationship. You will learn about each other and probably also learn more about yourself in the process.

There are two prerequisites for games of imaginative sex: affection and trust. You will open yourself up to another, revealing some of your deepest feelings and desires. That requires a high level of trust. The nature of some of these games require trust for the maximum comfort level. If you do not trust you partner, nervousness and fear could detract from benefits of imaginative sex. Think about the bondage aspects especially. Would you trust this person with $5000 of your money? If the answer is no, then why would you let them tie you up and gag you? As a romantic, I also believe that love will derive from these games as a natural consequence of the experience.

There is also a need for equality between men and women within these adventures. Women are not seen as inferior beings, simply as different people with their own strengths. If one partner is passive, or does not understand, or does not join in fully, these games are impossible. A woman's ideas, her inventions, her imaginations are as necessary and as important as those of the man. Passivity will only ruin the games and thwart their objectives. Both partners need to take an active role, even if one is the more submissive. As one famous fantasy author wrote "A girl who is bold is likely to think of marvels of pleasure for her master which a more timid girl would not dare to even contemplate."

Discussing Sexual Fantasies

How can we possibly know what erotic fantasies are going on inside a lover's head unless we ask them? Many women will assume that men fantasise about strippers and pole dancers but just because those are popular media images, it does not mean that most men are thinking about such things. I for one, find that strippers leave me cold and my own fantasies are far more complex and unusual. Women are even less predictable. Try asking one, "What makes construction workers so sexy?" and it is unlikely she will be able to tell you. We think that we are very well-versed in what the opposite sex finds sexy and why, but that is not always the case.

Women's fantasies are as wide and varied as women themselves. Of course, there are perennial favourites: the bad boy, the man in uniform, the brooding Celt. Some involve a college professor or a man in uniform but what it is about these images that are so arousing. Simply discussing such subjects can trigger a whole lot of fun in the bedroom. Unfortunately, some women are often embarrassed to talk about any of their imagined scenarios. Women have been raised not to speak up, expecting the man to read their minds and figure out what to touch, how to do so, and all without a GPS. Try to let go of the guilt. You can always preface your conversation with "This is hard for me to tell you because it makes me feel squeamish and embarrassed, but sometimes I fantasize about...."

Most women can be reassured that even in their day-to-day lives they have constant role shifts and daydreaming/fantasizing occurs all the time. She is a wife, a mother, a daughter, and an accountant. All of these require her to assume different behaviours. And chances are that she daydreams about something she would like to physically have, that vacation trip, new car, house etc. So if they can do it in daily public life why would it not happen as naturally in their private intimate lives?

Most likely you will find that your honesty (and an active imagination) is a major turn on. Be sincere. You should not be ashamed of what gets you off. Your partner is there to help you have fun in a protected and private environment. Do not think in terms of having kinks or weird fetishes. Think of your fantasies as part of your sex speciality; something unique that you can bring to the sexual experience. If you are feeling shy then practice saying the fantasy out loud. This might sound tedious but if you are not used to talking dirty or sharing your fantasies, then it is a good idea to have a few practice runs; that way you will not feel tongue tied when it comes time to share. Test the waters. During your next sexual encounter, say to your lover, "Want to hear my naughty fantasy?"

If you want your partner to feel comfortable fulfilling your sexual fantasy why not ask about theirs and offer to help out. Sharing your fantasies will encourage her to open up. She will feel comfortable talking to you in no time. However, do not share everything in an instant. Do it slowly. Look at her reactions before you continue with the details. A woman has to trust the person for her to share things she never thought she would ever reveal. These are her greatest secrets and she only wants to discuss them with someone she feels comfortable with. Tell her that you are an open-minded individual. Tell her that you do not mind exploring sexual fantasies. Women like to share their fantasies to guys who are open-minded and who will not judge them. Knowing her sexual desires is important if you want to have a great sex life. Guys have to be aware of what their lovers want. Do not make assumptions. Even if she loves the sex, she will always dream about her fantasies and hope that someday you will satisfy her desires. Do not wait for her to lose interest in you. Let her open up to you. Once she tells you her darkest secrets, be sure to make them come true.

Men have more permission to fantasize for two key reasons. Male masturbation is a much more common occurrence and most have had more experience a lot more porn material, both of which are enhanced by personalizing the experience with a fantasy. This means that they learn from the get go they have to use their minds to create more sensation and they learn how to do so almost immediately.

It has been said that a man's porn preferences are a true window to his soul. Just as the kind of porn that a man prefers is extremely revealing about his sexual tastes, asking a woman her sexual fantasy is a new way of saying, "Who are you?" If she tells you, she may be doing a mental strip-tease or she may be trying to liberate herself. Certainly she is taking a candid look at herself, because revealing one's sexual fantasies means opening up a very intimate and hitherto very repressed part of herself. A man's interest can be very helpful in discreetly inquiring, inspiring, and discerning these unspoken desires. It creates a more intimate connection and helps to shed taboos. In many cases there are often unexpected benefits. I clearly recall confessing to one girlfriend that I wanted to have sex with a girl while another girl held her down. I was delighted to learn that her fantasy was to be the girl holding her down.

Men will usually be relieved to learn that women's fantasies do not always involve steroid-induced bulges or even the most banging' bods.

Much more important in getting her pulse racing are long penetrating gazes and the flashing fire of intelligence in a man's eyes. Wouldn't it be revealing if for once at the climax of a beauty pageant, the three finalists were each in turn asked to answer the question, "What is your deepest, darkest, most secret fantasy?" An even better question might be "What would be the one thing you'd like try if you knew it was going to be the last fuck of your entire life?"

If your lover confides in you their deepest, darkest desires, respect the trust that they have in you. If they seize up, do not take it personally. Often introducing something new makes people feel they are sexually inadequate and will put them on the defensive. If they are not comfortable sharing their fantasy, do not pressure them. Respect their reaction. If they do not want to hear then you need to pull back and move on. If you can persuade your partner to open up, do not promise not to get mad, and then proceed to get mad. If your boyfriend confesses "I dream about your sister." or "I like to look at anime porn." remember that they are just fantasies.

Everyone has different standards for what is kinky. Communication will make it all better. Start small, go slow. Successfully integrating new ideas into your regular love making routine need to be brought in gently. If you approach your partner with a costume, script or whip you will most likely get shut down. Start by telling them you had a wild dream and that they were in it. If you approach it that way you can avoid making them feel like you are not satisfied with your lovemaking. Start by letting your partner know there is something you would love to try with 'THEM'. To heighten the idea, you might consider starting this conversation in the morning or when you are not in the bedroom. That gives your imagination more time to build up anticipation. Also name your source as that is likely going to be your partner's first question, "What brought this up?" Maybe it was a steamy scene in a film, some erotic literature or something that you have done before with a new and added twist. Introduce one idea at a time. Once you are clear about what feeling you want to produce, choose one at most two ways to initially try things out. If you try to include every idea at once it will dilute the intensity of the fantasy.

Allow your partner to help plan the fantasy, whether it is an adult DVD, lingerie or taboo location, let her make suggestions and participate in the discussions. You will find that when they help with the game plan that the result will be amazing. If your partner is uncomfortable with regular pornography, suggest a sex-education video. It will be tamer than porn and you could even pick up a new position or two. Try to use the tools available to you. Reading aloud passages from erotica is a good opener. It can be much easier when the words you are saying are not your own. Another option is to act out a sexy scene from your favourite movie. This is often easier since the template is already in place. A friend of mine went online and ordered two books of erotic short stories for women, and then downloaded them to them to his wife's Kindle. While she was away on a business trip, she wrote to him that she had found the books, and had been reading them. One particular story, she said, was driving her crazy. In a good way of course. She had been on the verge of going blind from the self passion that she had been enjoying from that particular story. When she arrived home, my friend was invited to read the story in bed, and act out the steamiest parts. It turned out to be the most heated session of their entire relationship.

Erotic role play helps improve communication with your partner. You get to learn each other's private sex fantasies and turn-ons, and then provide them, pleasurably. What a delicious gift to give each other. And never forget — this is play! Grown-up games are the best and sexiest kind.

Getting Your Fantasy Started

Stop dreaming about the best sex you have never had. It is time to start having the best sex you will ever have. Fantasies do not mean you are weird or kinky and there is no reason anybody should be offended. Make a sexual fantasy list and put them in proper order. The ones that are easy to fulfil come first. Think about location, costs, clothing, materials, music and how many people you want to involve.

Think about a suitable time. Some fantasies can last one night, some only a few minutes. For fantasies that are longer and involve visiting other places for a 'sexual trip' you should schedule your time. Grab a calendar and choose the dates when you can be totally immersed in these activities.

Halloween is the perfect time to 'go public' with a fantasy—as everyone is expecting you to dress up and act differently anyway. Many couples report that Halloween has turned into their favourite holiday because they can completely let loose; that the build-up of adventurous energy leads to amazing sex.

Know the difference between fantasy sexual role play and dirty talk. Having a few minutes of dirty talk just before you start having sex is not the same as setting out a fantasy role play scene. Role play can take you deeper into another character and release you from the restrictions you put on yourself in your daily life. It means more preparation, and more risks, but the difference is palpable, and worth it!

Great fantasy sexual role play requires some forethought. Most people start out a bit shy and nervous with the idea of dressing up as someone else and playing a role. Much of this reticence comes from a lack of preparation. The best way to get comfortable with sexual role playing is to get prepared. It is hard to leap into action (and a loin cloth) if you have never thought about how Tarzan might sound, or what he might want to do with Jane, and all those vines.

Consider the following elements of any sex role play scenario:

Who do you want to be? Pick a fantasy sexual role that feels right. It is hard to play a cliché that has no personal meaning, so find one that fits. It is fantasy and you can push your boundaries while finding a character that you connect with in some way.

What is the scenario? Details can take you deeper into a sexual role play scenario. When you first imagine a sexual scene the main points may be enough to get you going, but the more detail you can add to the fantasy the more alive it becomes. Even if you keep them to yourself, thinking through details can also be great for awkward moments when you do not know what to do next.

How can you dress it up? Maybe the most fun part of the preparation is costumes. As adults we do not get to play nearly enough, and fantasy sexual role play is a perfect opportunity to dress up and have fun. Once you have decided on who you want to be, think about ways to add to your character and role through clothing and props.

What is your motivation? Analyse your fantasy sexual role play character. Now that you know who you are, where you are, and what you are wearing, it is time to consider the psychology of your role. Analyse your character. What is your motivation? What turns your character on, what turns them off, what pushes their buttons or drives them wild? Are you dominant? Submissive? Do you switch back and forth?

What are the boundaries? Set ground rules for fantasy sexual role play. Setting ground rules and boundaries with the person or people you are going to be playing out a fantasy sexual role play with is essential. Some of these rules should be common sense and common courtesy, like no laughing at someone, and no judging each other in the moment. Other rules will take some thought and good communication.

Practice makes perfect. Use masturbation to explore fantasy sexual role play. When we think of sexual fantasies we usually imagine it involves at least two people. But masturbation offers some of the most fertile ground for developing sexual fantasy scenes. When we are masturbating we are less likely to censor our thoughts and feelings. It is all about sensation, sensuality, and intimacy.

The Beginner's Guide To Sexploration

Everyone fantasizes to one extent or another. For some, the fantasies are rather plain and simple while others compose very elaborate scenarios. Imaginative sex allows us to indulge our naughty side and act out our fantasies, turning them into sexual role-playing scenarios. In these scenarios, we can create different characters. We can envision ourselves and our partners as entirely different people. Costumes can be created to enhance the effect while props or decorations can be used to make the effect even more intense. Even so, these are not an absolute necessity. The human mind is so powerful that absolutely anything can be imagined.

Sexual role play is an exciting way for you and your partner to step out of your ordinary erotic routine and add a dash of spice to your love life. Take this opportunity to pretend to be someone else – your sexier, super-suave alter ego perhaps, or your more innocent younger self. Sometimes you might have a long-held favourite sex fantasy in mind, but other times you might be looking for inspiration. For those moments when you are ready to experiment, we have plenty of suggested scenarios to whet your imagination. Do not worry about how good an actor or actress you are. The point is not to win an Academy Award – it is to entice and seduce your very willing partner in sexual passion. They are your lover, not your critic; that means they have an ulterior motive to overlook any stumbling, hesitation, or blushing on your part. Remember, they probably also feel much the same way. Keep it light and fun and you will be fine.

Wait until you are both really turned on. You will likely underestimate your boundaries if you try to talk about them when you are in your cold state. This is why revealing your fantasies when you are in the heat of passion is such a good idea; both of you will be so hot and bothered that things which normally freak you out actually sound quite reasonable and, dare I say it, sexy. No matter how bizarre or incomprehensible, these fantasies reveal something intimate about a person's personality and psychological functioning. It has been suggested that a person who craves attention might repetitively fantasize about being the centre attraction at an orgy, whereas another who has deep-seated feelings of guilt might fantasize about being sexually punished and humiliated. The key trigger for arousal in these sexual fantasies is where the fantasy resonates, like a tuning fork, with the existing elements of the person's personality. Even so, there is no relationship between disturbing and complex, fantastic sexual fantasies, and any level of mental disturbance. Sexual fantasizing can be healthy, particularly for a reasonably healthy couple that uses their increased excitement to move toward rather than away from the partner.

Some of our own more extreme fantasies and thoughts may frighten and even disturb us but that does not mean that they need to be acted upon. They are not burning desires that must be satiated, they are simply fantasies. Research shows that surprisingly large levels of socially-unacceptable, frightening and and often disturbing fantasies live inside the heads of the normal people around us. And yet the amounts of infidelity, incest, bestiality, group sex and other behaviours, going on every day are actually very low in frequency. They are very normal as fantasies, and in the vast majority of cases, remain fantasies. Fear of rejection and stigma leads people to keep these fantasies secret from everyone, often even their wives, husbands and therapists. Most people believe they are the only ones with such fantasies, but this is rarely the case. In fact, the average person's mind contains so much diversity and complexity, that speaking about a 'normal' fantasy is almost meaningless.

The fantasy of the 'threesome' with two women is regarded as ubiquitous among men, with some prevalence rates as high as 85% of males acknowledging such a fantasy. It is such a common a fantasy that no one regards it as strange, but simply sees it as "normal." But how many men actually have such sexual experiences? Fewer than 6%. Men are happy to talk about their fantasies. Well, some men, and most fantasies, particularly if it is a fantasy figure – a celebrity, for example, with whom they enjoy imagining a sexual liaison. Men are much more likely to fantasize about having threesomes or orgies. In general, men respond to the visual. Fast. Men also respond to scent. A lingering fragrance left on a pillow can conjure intense emotions, and strong physical reactions. Male fantasies tend to focus more on visual imagery and explicit anatomic detail, whereas women's fantasies tend to contain more emotion and connection. Women can respond to a visual stimulus, including the beauty of other women. They also respond to the pleasures of the male form – just not necessarily as much, or as quickly. A woman's' timing is different. Women percolate, while men come to a quick boil. They do not usually go from zero to sixty in ten seconds flat.

Wigs and costumes can be a big help towards getting into character. An authentic-looking police uniform can make frisking come more naturally to you. Even a simple wig could be enough to make you feel uncharacteristically saucy. If you are turned off by the idea of having a sit-down planning session, Halloween or a costume party might the perfect opportunity to slip into role playing. Take charge of the costumes you will both be wearing. Then keep those costumes on when you get home and make your move. The role-playing will come much more naturally then.

It might help to realise that we live in a a culture based on fantasy and acting out. For boys the mock gunfights of childhood soon turn into adolescent war games. Video gamers becomes a space pilots trying to save the universe or soldiers in a combat simulations. Girls act out the role of parent ministering to a doll that acts as a surrogate child. Toys provide a kind of symbolic arena, and are used as props, which allow children to lose themselves in the dramas of play, acting out issues that are central to their stage of development. As we grow older our role-playing takes a more passive role but remains just as common place. Television, movies and theatre allow us to identify with fictional characters. The murder mystery allows us to take on the role of detective, solving the crime and defending the moral order of society. We are regularly taken for wild rides in amusement parks and on roller coasters. These are all examples of role plays or simulations. If anything, role play is so common place in our normal lives, it seems a little strange that more people do not do it in the bedroom.

Some people might enjoy writing down their fantasies. The prototype here, though more extensive and developed, would be the 'director's play book,' in which the director has not only the script, but his notes, stage directions, sketches of scenery, costumes, etc. This challenges the idea that it is the coolest characters in our society that make the best lovers. The reality is that in many cases the most physically attractive are little more than vases, beautiful to look at but not much inside. The shocking truth may well be that the geeks and the nerds turn out to be the best lovers. They are the ones that are most able to stimulate the brain, every individuals important sexual organ. They are the ones with the most experience and practical skill in gaming, role playing and story telling. In a long term relationship, an imaginative geek beats a bimbo or a beefcake every time.

Remember, the first few times you try adding fantasy to your lovemaking, there are bound to be screw ups. Give it some time before it feels comfortable. After a while fantasy-inspired sex will be times to look forward to. When the endorphins have settled, do a follow-up. After the sex, ask how they liked it and would like to do it again.

FIFTY FANTASIES

1. ALIEN ENCOUNTERS

Science fiction is the fastest growing film and literary genre in the world today and so futuristic fantasies have become a staple of sexual role play. What self-respecting geek has never imagined himself as Captain Kirk in a harem of Orion sex slaves or seducing an alien princess as part of an important diplomatic mission? An alien fantasy need not necessarily mean being dragged into the bushes, tasered, and forcibly anally probed by tentacled monsters. Unless of course, you are Japanese, in which case it might even be obligatory.

As alien fantasies become ever more popular, a whole industry is springing up around sci-fi sexuality. The Alien Cathouse, a sci-fi themed whorehouse has recently opened its doors, just down the highway from the notorious Area 51 top-secret UFO facility in Nevada. Futuristically themed rooms and girls in Princess Leia costumes are proving to be a popular draw. For solo play, a bizarre and confusing Avatar-themed blue "Alien" flesh-light male masturbation unit is available in sex shops. There is even a terrifying alien dildo available for those wanting a genuine xenomorphallus experience. The Mythos is eleven inches long and two inches across (not around – across!). This monster is frightening in the way that it pushes psychological and biological boundaries.

There has always been an strong undercurrent in science fiction. Some film critics for example have proposed that the classic H. R. Giger Alien is a horrific display of phallic power. A giant erection - complete with teeth and dripping with semen-like ooze - shoots out of the Alien's mouth to penetrate the flesh of its victims. The same film also features Ripley's air lock strip-tease, featuring thong-like panties and a luridly voyeuristic ensconcement into her space suit. It was as if Ridley Scott suddenly decided that a little hormonal teenage T&A was needed after the dark, mature horror. The finale of Alien took place in the tight quarters of the shuttle Narcissus where Sigourney Weaver performs a strip tease for the audience, shedding the plain green jumpsuit that had masked her sexuality throughout the film. Her nipples stood erect under a tight-fitting white tank top, the last of three layers that had hidden her female shape. Her bottom half was bare and her panties were two sizes too small and cut so low as to reveal much more that we would normally expect. A strobe light effect pervades the mise-en-scene, titillating the audience as if Ripley were participating in a pornographic photo shoot. The alien's arm pops out, catching the distracted audience off guard having been lulled into a voyeuristic gaze. She hides in a storage area and the objective camera fetishizes her body, looking her up and down from a low angle that emphasizes her sexy curves.

Seductive characters fill the torrent of science fiction films and novels that have been released in the last two decades. My own personal favourites include Zotoh Zhaan from the Australian TV series Farscape, Neytiri in James Cameron's Avatar, and Liara Ts'oni in the Mass Effect video game series. Literary fans might well recognize Gena Showalter's fantastic Alien Huntress series, where Devyn, King of the Targons, is a warrior, a womaniser and perhaps the hottest alien ever. Science fiction is filled with inspiration for fantasy scenarios.

Many women harbour these strange and exotic fantasies. These range from being captured and imprisoned by monster aliens and being treated as a sex pet, tentacle raped, and having their will and mind broken to being made pregnant with a cross-breed child, or their bodies surgically altered so that they can carry their species offspring.

To quote one internet poster:

"I want to be fucked into insanity, nothing more than prey for them to do what they will. They will eventually either be too rough or get bored with me, then they'll tear me apart and eat me as they should have done at the start. Or maybe they would prefer to keep me around for milking and spawning purposes. They use me like a human uses a cow, but for their own perverse interspecies lust as well. I am degraded and dominated with a huge case of Stockholm syndrome. If I'm a good girl they might even think of me affectionately, as a true pet and not a prisoner. If I'm a bad girl they can replace me easily and kill me. The idea of being raped by something physically strange and repulsive is basically instant wetness for me. I'm not a zoophile, but I get really horny about the idea of being dominated and used by another kind of creature, the more terrifying and exotic the better! I would willingly sacrifice myself to be Cthulu's abomination spawner!"

Whenever I run a fantasy narrative for my own partner, I always describe the alien captor as decidedly humanoid but almost superhuman in his physical attributes. What follows is an example of the way in which I excite her verbally, having her close her eyes and conjure up visions to accompany my lurid description.

"I want you to picture a huge blue-skinned man. Not just any man, a man sculpted and honed by the harsh environment of an alien world. Not some freaky Charles Atlas caricature or Arnold Schwarzenegger wannabe but something even stronger, something beyond human, something super human. Even though he is clearly not human, he is a larger-than-life symbol of everything that is male. He is a walking testosterone warrior. His build is that of a concrete dam, with shoulders as broad as battlements, and with more abs than you can possibly count. His chest is hairless and smooth, only a slowly widening trail leading from his belly button down into his pubic hair, already soaked and matted in sweat and pheromones. His interstellar penis is not anything a human could aspire to. It fills you with awe. It is a towering pillar of flesh, with features that will drive you wild once inside you. Thick bulging veins and an angry a flaring head. Beneath it are two colossal, smooth orbs, visibly churning with his seed, in a dark, tight sack that cannot possibly hold them.

And speaking of his seed, the first sign of pre-cum is leaking out of the tip. You can smell it. It is a rich, delicious aroma, very different to

17

that of human men. It has a smell that is both repugnant and alluring at the same time. It is a gross sticky ooze but beneath that, it is an ambrosia and you yearn to feel it on your tongue. You want to taste it. You crave it. Your body burns for it. You know, without any doubt, that if you wrap your lips around that head, truly there is no going back, you will be his slave forever. You will not be able to go a single night without him and without aching for his hot seed. You will be tortured by the feeling of emptiness in the holes that will be carved out by his monstrous alien member, unsatisfied save for those wonderful times that he is deep inside you.

The first beads of his alien sperm are dribbling down his thick pulsating shaft. A solitary bead begins to well up and fall to the ground. It pains you to think even of a drop of his precious seed will be wasted, and you lunge forward to catch it on your tongue. Slowly, deliberately you let that heavenly nectar make its warm way down your throat. It tastes awful and amazing at the very same time. You want to gag but you also feel warm inside. Within a moment your tongue is sliding up along the bottom of his shaft, slurping up the rest of the spilled liquid. You know you need to feel this deep inside you and so you set to work.

Later, much, much later, he tosses you aside, bubbling spunk oozing from every hole. You know he does not care about you. You were just a warm, wet, eager set of holes. And it does not matter, because you know are just an earthling sex toy to him, moulded to his body, needing his seed in your belly to feel complete."

My own background means that I am quite an accomplished story teller and so I can have a fast and powerful effect on my partners. If you are still developing these skills then maybe start with a simpler description.

Of course, the alien need not always be a super human alpha male. It might instead be an interplanetary monster. Men are not the only things females are sexually curious about. In this fantasy, the nature of the monster is, of course, up to the female. If she is to be violated, she should certainly have something to say about its appearance. Perhaps it is mammalian in nature but it is obviously alien. Perhaps it is very large and covered with silken fur, maybe with several prehensile appendages. It is doubtless extremely strong. Its mouth is an enormous jaw filled with sharp teeth that could easily bite through an entire shoulder of hers, if it chose. The eyes are the huge dark discs of a nocturnal predator. Unlike earth creatures, it might be of even greater intelligence than human beings. Perhaps it captures her and takes her, gently, in its mouth, and carries her, on four feet, in loping strides, to its den. There it drops her on grasses and soft mosses and, perhaps with its teeth, strips her. When it holds her, in its several furred, prehensile appendages, she is completely helpless. She cannot move. There is no escape for her. It bends more closely to her. She turns her head to one side. She smells its fur, its odors. She sees the large eyes. She feels its powerful, silken, furred grasp. She hears it breathing. She screams, as it penetrates her.

An alien lover need not always be male of course. There are always a very wide range of female characters to provide you with inspiration. Some of these are now a part of our societies cultural fabric, such as Princess Leia in her chains and slave girl outfit. The role of alien princess can very easily be recognisably humanoid. She might be the alluring Aurora, evil, sadistic daughter of Ming the Merciless from the Flash Gordon tales. At the other end of the scale she might be a intergalactic damsel in distress figure, a defenceless waif that you have rescued from space pirates. She need not have green skin or two heads. Such excesses are best left to the Hollywood special effects wizards and body painting parties. For my own part, I find that a simple pair of forehead mounted feathery antenna are more than enough to convince me that I have an authentic alien on my hands. They attach very easily with a little water-based make-up glue or can be purchased as part of a budget Halloween costume. It is surprising how alien princesses bear a striking resemblances to fantasy princesses from earth literature. To this end, any belly dancing outfit would be suitable for creating a convincing costume. Diaphanous silks and baggy satin pants might sound more like Arabian Nights than alien world, but they certainly do the trick.

The incredible growth of cosplay means that there are now more costumes available then ever before. It has never been easier to transform yourself into a everything from a Victorian time traveller to a rampaging space marine. A quick change of clothes allow anybody to boldly go where no man has gone before, exploring distant galaxies in the comfort of your own bedroom. Exotic alien weapons make for some very interesting S&M situations. Klingon ceremonial daggers add a new dimension to kidnap scenarios as do blasters and exotic laser pistols. I personally like to have some Ozric Tentacles or similarly psychedelic music playing in the background for added extra-terrestrial effect.

Due to the limits of TV and film special effects, many of us are quite limited in our ideas about aliens. Even now with complex CGI most alien species are kept surprisingly similar to our own, in order to appeal to the widest audience possible. Although the Daphne Guinness music video for 'Evening In Space' was an refreshing exploration of interspecies sex, most formulaic action movies require the same boring shoot-outs and so alien differences are rarely explored in any real detail. The same is not true for science fantasy literature, and I would urge you to be adventurous in your reading in order to expand your imagination in this area. A good starting point might be the pacifist space operas of James White. Sector General is a series of twelve science fiction novels set in the Sector 12 General Hospital, a huge hospital space station located in deep space, designed to treat a wide variety of life forms with a wide range of ailments and life-support requirements, and to house an equally diverse staff. The series is noted for its diverse and believable non-humanoid alien life forms.

2. Animal Encounters

Your wild erotic nature may emerge in animal fantasies. Do not worry, having animal sex fantasies does not (usually) mean you want to have sex with animals in real life. You may just revel in the ultra-taboo, bestial wildness. Horses and dogs figure commonly in men's bestiality fantasies which usually involve them submissively receiving sex from the animal or voyeuristically watching a woman engaged in sex with the animal. Female fantasies tend to involve the woman being the animal, often something in the wild "pussy" family, such as a lioness, tiger or cheetah. No wonder wildcat patterns are so popular in women's fashion.

Of course, real-life bestiality is appalling to most people. But animal sex fantasies connect you to your animal nature, often freeing your mind from the all-too-human sexual oppression that lurks within you. It was not so long ago that any form of sexuality not leading to the conception of children was seen as, at best, wanton lust, or worse, a perversion and a sin. One by one, those taboos have fallen. In many of the world's great cities, gays and lesbians can be open about their sexual preferences to an extent unimaginable a century ago. Oral sex? Some objected to President Clinton' choice of place and partner, but no one dared suggest that he was unfit to be President simply because he had enjoyed a blow job.

Of course, not every taboo has crumbled. Sex with animals is still definitely taboo but this might not be because of its rarity. Midas Dekkers, a Dutch biologist, popular naturalist and author of Dearest Pet, has shown that humans have often thought of "love for animals" in ways that go well beyond a pat and a hug. His book has a wide range of illustrations, going back to a Swedish rock drawing from the Bronze Age of a man penetrating a large quadruped of indeterminate species. There is a Greek vase from 520 BC showing a male figure having sex with a stag. A seventeenth-century Indian miniature of a deer mounting a woman. The Roman mythological tradition is filled with sexual encounters between humans and animals, especially mortal women and gods in the guise of animals. Most famous are the stories of Jupiter (Greek Zeus), who visits Leda as a swan and Europa as a bull. And the the Minotaur born of Pasiphaë and a bull. Satyrs, known for their sexual voracity, are often pictured with bestial features. An eighteenth-century European engraving of an ecstatic nun coupling with a donkey, while other nuns look on, smiling. A nineteenth-century Persian painting of a soldier, also with a donkey and, from the same period, a Japanese drawing of a woman enveloped by a giant octopus who appears to be sucking her to ecstasy, as well as caressing her body with its many limbs.

Non-sexual animal role-play, or therianthropy, was a common and integral part of ritual in many tribal cultures both in recent and likely prehistoric times, where members of the tribe would take the role physically and often spiritually of an animal that was either revered or hunted. Examples of the former include many of the American Indian tribes and Arctic native peoples. It is also sometimes used in education, especially physical education, as a way to encourage people to exercise the body in unusual ways, by mimicking various animals. Many of the most effective forms of Chinese Kung Fu are animal based forms.

In the 1940s, Kinsey asked twenty thousand Americans about their sexual behaviour, and found that eight percent of males and 3.5 percent of females stated that they had, at some time, had a sexual encounter with an animal. Among men living in rural areas, the figure shot up to fifty percent. Dekkers suggests that for young male farm hands, animals provided an outlet for sexual desires that could not be satisfied when girls were less willing to have sex before marriage. They may also take advantage of the sucking reflex of calves to get them to do a blow job. When I was at college, one fellow student confessed that he coated his cock in dried fish food and let the giant koi carp in his Dad's pond nibble him to climax.

For three-quarters of the women who told Kinsey that they had had sexual contact with an animal, the animal involved was a dog, and actual sexual intercourse was rare. More commonly the woman limited themselves to touching and masturbating the animal, or having their genitals licked by it. I once dated a girl who told me that, when she and her sister were teenagers, they had let their childhood dog lick peanut butter off their vaginas until they orgasmed. It was many years later that I dated her, and by that time she had developed extremely elaborate werewolf fantasies. Girls are far more likely to be attracted to horses than boys, and sitting with legs astride a rhythmically moving horse undoubtedly has a sexual undertone. Dekkers agrees, adding that "the horse is the ideal consolation for the great injustice done to girls by nature, of awakening sexually years before the boys in their class, who are still playing with their train sets . . . "

Most would argue that bestiality should be illegal, at least in in so far as it shows cruelty towards an animal. Some acts are clearly wrong, and should remain crimes. The practice of some men using a hen as a sexual object, inserting their penis into the cloaca, the all-purpose back channel is usually fatal to the hen, and in some cases she will be deliberately decapitated just before ejaculation in order to intensify the convulsions of its sphincter. This is cruelty, clear and simple. And yet, who has not been at a social occasion disrupted by the household dog gripping the legs of a visitor and giving them a vigorous humping? The host usually discourages such activities, but in private not everyone objects to such an activity.

As far as I am concerned, only consenting partners should be considered acceptable. There are many bizarre and unusual fantasies in this book but the one strand that binds then all together is that every act is consensual, even the non-consent rape fantasies. To this end I would like to suggest a number of scenarios that involve humans acting as animals, rather than actual members of a different species.

The first of these is the two animal fantasy, whereby a male and female animal encounter one another, and mate. A large number of very young children fantasize about birds, fish, cows, and many other species mating with each other, long before they have any sexual awakenings of their own.

In this scenario, two animals, without speech, who have never encountered one another, and have never had sexual relations, meet. The animals are human animals, but still animal. They know nothing of sex, but, strangely, they feel attracted to one another. They smell one another, they study one another; they circle one another; they growl, warning one another off; they whine, inviting the other's closer approach. They rub timidly against one another, and find it pleasurable. They touch one another, and kiss and lick one another. Soon, driven by their instincts, they mate. They are then companions, inseparable.

This can be a beautiful fantasy, and is useful for teaching human beings the loving body. It is important in this fantasy to really feel oneself as an animal, relating to another animal. It helps human beings, often too cerebral, too complex, too abstract, too ready to conceptualize, meet one another on a level almost of pure attraction and instinct. The animal in man is beautiful, and this fantasy helps to celebrate it. There are many animals to choose from each one with different physical attributes and sensations. Dogs and cats are clearly very different but something that many people can relate to. More imaginative partners might want to try and put themselves in the role of a boar and sow. This could even be extrapolated all the way up to a rhinoceros or a hippopotamus. Chimps are great fun and very different to large predators such as lions and tigers. Cow play often involves fantasies of lactation and impregnation.

An interesting alternative is the male livestock fantasy, whereby herds of men are kept by oversized, alien females. They are controlled with signals, with whips, and alien dog-like creatures who drive them back to their stalls at night, where they are locked in. In the morning and the evening they are "milked." Their semen furnishes the large women with energy. They are "milked" on their backs, with the large females kneeling across their bodies. After their morning use they are driven out to the pasture; after their evening use they are returned to their stalls. To the aliens they are only animals, and are bought and sold, and bred as such. They are always naked. Animals do not wearclothing, although members of an owner's herd can be marked with a distinguishing device.

Another variant of the dominant female role here is that the woman is capable of physically intimidating and abusing the male into compliance. She can order him to serve her in any way she pleases. She holds his head, by the hair, between her legs for hours, until she is satisfied, not releasing him perhaps until she has been carried through a lengthy series of delicious, fantastic orgasms. Then, at last, perhaps weary, she might, rape him before sending him back to his kennel for the night.

Human pony play is a form of role-play where one person acts like a pony or horse, while their partner takes on the role of rider, trainer or caretaker. It is also known as equus eroticus (Latin), particularly in femdom circles. Pony play is traditionally done with female submissives but works just as well for male submissives. The submissive is treated as a "pony," and fairly elaborate scenario can be constructed around the buying of a new pony, the humiliating rituals of checking teeth and genitals for health problems, and the teaching and learning of new gaits and tricks. For example, the dominant can stand still with a crop, with the submissive on a tether (attached to a bit or even to nipple piercings), and have the submissive run in circles around the dominant until he or she reaches a constant speed for 'walk', for 'canter', for 'gallop', and so on. The crop can be used for 'motivation', "Get those knees up!" for example. For this type of pony play is that all you really need are a bit gag, some rope for reins, a 'hitching post', and space. A variant on this is adding a 'pony tail' (a fall of hair attached to a butt plug) which can be fun to comb, to braid, and even to tie bows in.

There are generally three kinds of pony"

Cart ponies: ponies who pull a sulky with their owner.

Riding ponies: ponies who are ridden, either on all fours or on two legs, with the "rider" on the shoulders of the "pony" (also known as Shoulder riding). Note that a human back is generally not strong enough to take the weight of another adult without risk of injury, so four-legged "riding" is generally symbolic, with the "rider" taking most of their weight on their own legs.

Show ponies: ponies who show off their dressage skills and often wear elaborate harnesses, plumes and so on.

The limited evidence that is available suggests that the fantasy and practice may be somewhat more prevalent in the U.K. than the U.S.A., which may be a reflection of the number of people familiar and used to ponies and horses. An endless array of bit gags, bridles, saddles, tack (harnesses), whips, butt plugs with tails, "hooves" that are worn like boots (sometimes also as gloves), and related items are produced and sold commercially to those who wish to act out such fantasies. A documentary film 'Pony Passion' was produced by the British pony play club De Ferre in 2003 showing their club's activities, and 'Born in a Barn' a 2005 documentary film, depicted the lives of several pony-play enthusiasts. National Geographic produced a documentary on the subject and there is another featuring Pony Play at Frolicon 2012. Some of the earliest published images of animal play (especially pony play) are to be found in the work of John Willie, primarily in Bizarre magazine published from 1948 to 1959. The first commercial manifestation of this fetish was created by Simon Benson, the founder of the Petgirls website. Peter Shaffer's 1973 play Equus tells the story of a young man who has a pathological religious fascination with horses, but this appears closer to zoophilia than pet play. One group, the LA Ponies and Critters Club, takes the community idea of BDSM animal role-play further by staging a mock fox hunt in local forested areas. These events bring together pony players, puppy players and their respective humans for a cooperative, community bonding activity. One of the canine players volunteers to be the "fox" and marks a trail in the forest. The other puppy players form the pack of "hounds" that search out the fox and bark/howl to bring the pony players and their "riders" to capture the "fox".

Species dysphoria, the feeling that one's body is of the wrong species is common within the otherkin and therian communities. This is also a contributing factor of the 'Furry' fandom community. As with most forms of role-play, its uses include play and psychodrama. Animal role-play may also be found in BDSM contexts, where an individual may be subjected to humiliation by being treated as an animal. The activity is often referred to as pet play. For some enthusiasts this can become extreme

"It is not about having sex with the animal, more like the animal having sex with me and me being treated like an animal. I am very submissive as it is, so thinking about being forced into a kennel turns me on enough already, but add other animals to the mix and the thought drives me crazy. I would love for my master to order me to get a dog off with my mouth or to let it fuck me in the ass. I would love even more to be tied down on my hands and knees with my legs spread apart and then get raped in the ass by a dog. The combination of getting dominated, humiliated, and being treated as if I am nothing but another dog really turns me on. This fantasy is not limited to dogs either, they are just a good example to use."

There seems to be a growing trend among the BDSM scene in animal role-play, especially pup and kitten play. Playing the role of a pup or kitten is one of giving over complete control over to another, while the 'master or handler' expects only unconditional love and obedience from his/her animal. In puppy play, the participants acts out canine mannerisms and behaviours, which is sometimes associated with leather culture. The dominant role is taken by a "handler", "trainer", "master", or in the case of someone who still identifies as canine, an "alpha". The submissive may be considered a "pup" or a "dog". Unlike other forms of animal role-play, it is not uncommon for two or more pups to play together as equals, fight for dominance, or play where one is clearly the "alpha". Puppy play is often about being playful, mischievous, and instinctive. Many human puppies like to simplify their desires and motivations as they embrace the side of themselves that acts solely on instinct. A "puppy" who is "unowned" or "uncollared" can be referred to as a "stray".

In kitten play, a person dresses to resemble and assumes the mannerisms and character of a kitten, a characteristic of which is that it keeps some independence and, as part of the fantasy, might retaliate against the partner trying to tame him or her. In manga and anime, a relatively common character type is the "catgirl," often a thin teenage girl with cat ears, a tail, tiny fangs and a propensity for catlike affection or curiosity. Examples include Cat Girl Nuku Nuku, Pink from Dragon Pink and Ms. Furbottom's human form in Sgt. Frog, among others. Real-life costume play, or cosplay, of anime cat girls could be considered a form of pet play. Some superheroes, heroines, and villains also feature elements related to pet play; such as DC Comics' Wildcat, Catwoman, the Penguin and Vixen, Marvel's Tigra, Man-Wolf and Black Cat, or even Nastassja Kinski's Irena Gallier in the 1982 film Cat People (a remake of the 1942 Simone Simon film), and Miss Kitty from the Brendan Fraser movie Monkeybone.

3. ARISTOCRAT TO SLAVE

In the twenty first century our society has been transformed from a hereditary aristocracy, with rankings and titles to a 'plutocracy,' where we are now ruled by the rich. Princes and kings have been replaced by bankers and oligarchs. Totalitarian governments threaten the fragile and perhaps, tragically, evanescent flower of rational democracy.

Let us for a moment imagine instead that we progressed from barbarous feudalism to a benevolent aristocracy, which concerns itself, if only out of noblesse oblige, to look after the welfare of the lower orders. Let us also suppose that two of the most prestigious and powerful aristocratic families have become embroiled in a brutal power struggle. The losers are now being tried by the victors for treason (or perhaps if you want to make it shockingly realistic, terrorism.)

A former countess, barefoot, in a simple one-piece prison tunic and prisoner chains, currently stands before the bar of justice. She is officially stripped of her title and her rank. She is now no longer of the aristocracy. Court security strip her of her single garment.

The judge appraises her carefully . "Your body is certainly most suitable," he muses.

He offers her the choice of execution or slavery.

"Are you a slave to be spared, or an aristocrat destined for the execution chambers?"

"I am a slave," she whispers.

"Speak up for the court, slave," orders the judge.

"I am a slave," she says, clearly. A buzz courses through the courtroom. There is shock. Her statement is entered into the transcript of the proceedings.

"It was wrong," sternly reprimands the judge, "for a slave to have pretended to have been an aristocrat."

"Yes," she whispers.

"Speak up, slave, or I will have the court officers beat the truth out of you." orders the judge.

"Yes, it was wrong." she says, clearly.

"Is it not true," he demands, "that such behaviour should be punished?"

"Yes," she cries.

"And is it not true that you should be legally designated as a slave?"

"Yes," she weeps.

"Do you not beg then," he asks, "to be legally enslaved?"

"Yes," she weeps.

"Yes, what?" he demands, sternly.

"Yes... Master," she whispers.

"Speak so the court can hear you," commands the judge.

"Yes... Master, I beg to be enslaved" she says, loudly, clearly.

"Let this slave," decrees the judge, "be officially registered as a female in bondage; let her body wear the brand of servitude; and let her throat be encircled with the collar of the state."

She looks at him, in misery.

"And then," continues the judge, "let her, after being suitably trained in the duties of a female slave, be transmitted, with other service and recreational materials, to Pacific Outpost 5A." The gavel strikes three times.

The miserable woman, formerly an aristocrat, now a mere criminal, convicted of treason, destined for slavery, is led from the bar of justice. Her world has crumbled. At the door of the court, her arm held by the hand of the bailiff, she stops, and looks back, agonized, at the judge. But he does not notice her. His gavel strikes again.

"Next case," he orders. By the arm, the bailiff's hand upon it, the girl, naked, is led through the door from the court. The door closes behind her. The attention of the court is now on the next poor wretch.

Pacific Outpost 5A is the most remote of the civilization's facilities, previously an island internment camp for unfortunate refugees unable to reach Australia. She is conducted by camp guards to the chamber of enslavement. Little time is lost in such matters. By nightfall she will wear her brand and collar. In the morning her training will begin.

The imprinting of the mark and locking on of the collar is done immediately. Locked into the branding rack, seeing the white heat of the iron, she realise that there will never be any escape from her misfortune.

I have included the details of the above script as it can be strong and powerfully erotic when acted out. How you continue the fantasy is up to you but here are some useful pointers. The shock of being transformed from aristocrat to slave is a theme that should be built upon for maximum effect. This is especially true if your partner is well educated in the real world. Slave names change frequently, but simply addressing her as 'Slave' will have a strong and lasting impact. Let her imagine that there is little chance of escape from this remote island prison. And how do the rough soldiers of the facility take to her, a former aristocrat, now only a slave for their use? How do they treat her? How does she feel? And does she, to her misery, find herself responding to them, as only a slave girl to the touch of masters? What does this do to her self-image? Is character conflict created within her? Perhaps in the arms of one man she comes particularly to love her collar. What does this mean?

Perhaps, somehow, she does manage to escape, perhaps with a man who abducts her, perhaps there is a war, perhaps there is an attack on the outpost by aliens, etc. Perhaps all the humans at the post are captured and taken to another planet, etc. Many plots and situations can develop intelligently within a given context of background and characters.

4. BABY-MAKING

In modern westernised societies, it is now common for a couple to want to concentrate on their careers before going though the complicated and expensive process of parenthood. Others might prefer to adopt, while others still might prefer the idea of having a pet dog or cat rather than having to cope with a child. All of us are different and we all have different aims and goals in our lives. One thing that does connect every one of us though is our history as a species. For many hundreds of thousands of years we have bred successfully, creating endless new generations of humankind. Procreation therefore plays an important psychological role in sex even if you see it as a purely recreational activity.

Some couples are both terrified of accidental pregnancy and neither of them wants children anytime soon. Even so, the idea of procreation can be extremely stimulating, even if is not really intended. It can make for an extremely powerful fantasy that will really get your hormones pumping. Even when you are enjoying protected sex, I urge you to give it a try and see how strong the effects can be for both partners.

Try using the language of procreation and it will undoubtedly have a strong effect on your orgasmic intensity. She should be egging him on with phrases like the following:

"I want you to cum inside me."

"I want you to spill your seed in my pussy."

"I want to have your baby."

"Cum inside me, get me pregnant, knock me up."

He can reply with a wide variety of responses:

"I'm going to cum inside you; I want to get you pregnant."

"Do you want my baby? Do you want to have my kids? Tell me you want to have my baby!"

"I'm going to plant my seed in you!"

"Would you have my baby? If I got you pregnant, would you keep it? Say you'd keep it!"

There are many variations on these phrases.

In my own experience, the following works well. "So you want me be a daddy? So tell Daddy that you need it faster and harder and deeper baby."

This opens all kinds of dirty baby-daddy talk that add an almost pornographic element to sex. As one expert stated, if sex is not dirty, then you obviously ain't doing it right. It branches over into incest fantasies, which by their strictly taboo nature are extremely exciting. Try finishing by whispering in her ear, "I hope you are pregnant now. You will be mine forever. I will call you in a few weeks to learn the happy news."

Some enthusiasts call this the 'breeding fetish' and it often leads on to a semen fascination. I knew one woman who would spontaneously start screaming "Breed me, you big sexy bastard!" and it would get pretty rough, pretty quick. The problem for some guys is that when their lover comes out with their hot ideas of impregnation, it can run a little too close to the seriousness of having children. In the average man's head, one skirts dangerously close to the other. For others, just talking during sex is difficult. I had a very close friend who complained that a young lady I had introduced him to would ask him repeatedly if he loved just as he was reaching the point of orgasm. I asked him if her requesting him to call her a bitch and talk dirty to her would also be a problem. He said that would be no problem at all. This helped him to realise that his words were simply helping her to live out her fantasies. What we say in the throes of orgasm should not be taken at face value.

Some men actually enjoy the baby making fantasy and phone-sex industry workers report that the impregnation scenario is requested quite regularly. It can be extremely exciting when, during the height of passion, a lover wraps her legs around you and begs to be filled by you, in order to make her a real woman. In reality, when some women near ovulation they became insanely sexual. One friend confided that his wife was no longer interested in her own orgasm, but only having him ejaculate inside her. She would orgasm very strongly, but it was her husband climaxing that really set her off. At such times of high hormones she would come back for more again and again, doing every trick she could think of to get him hard again, and jumping him over and over. For a guy with high sex drive, this can be wonderful. Even though she was not usual a big fan of oral sex, she would repeatedly offer him blow jobs just to get him hard and then want him to finish inside her. Normally she would have resisted if he had been inside her without washing but at this time she did not care, she just wanted him hard again. If was if she had a one track mind and it was "Give me the sperm and then I will be happy."

5. BABYSITTERS, NANNIES AND GOVERNESSES

There is a very good chance that many readers have been babysitters at some point in their lives. Sometimes this was an undesirable and unpaid but entirely obligatory gig, watching a younger family member. For others it might have been the first example of paid employment that they were able to find. With so much personal experience tied up in the simple role of baby sitter, it is no wonder that it is such a rich vein of sexual fantasy from which we can draw.

Babysitting represents the very first financial and sexual independence of teenage girls. It is therefore almost inseparable from the transformation from adolescent innocent to sexually awakening young woman. The rise of the babysitter coincided with the rise of the teenage girl as a cultural phenomenon in the 1920s. Babysitting was a compromise between "teenage girls' desire for personal freedom and adults' expectations that they stay close to home. Ever since that time, there has been an endless stream of erotica centred on the sexy babysitter. At first these tales were a mainstay of x-rated novels and magazines but there are now literally thousands of movies about about super-sexy sitters. These range from mainstream slasher movies to hardcore porn based on adult male fantasies about the sexual willingness of teenage girls.

The nanny suggests feeling of comfort and safety and is often thought of as an older woman but this can still evoke thoughts of lust in many men, especially those who were left in the care of a nanny as a youngster. These days the nanny has morphed into the sexy, continental au-pair. The celebrity media is filled with stories of Hollywood stars that have left their wives for their nannies. Ethan Hawke left Uma Thurman for their nanny. Jude Law cheated on Sienna Miller with their nanny. Robin Williams married the nanny he and his first wife hired. Rob Lowe's former nanny allegedly had an affair with him.

Not to mention Tiger Woods' marriage to his former nanny. Experts claim that it is all related to them falling for the nurturing personality. Nannies already know their homes and provide a sexy comfort that busy wives forget.

Long before babysitters, there were extensive cultural anxieties about the sexual availability of governesses. It was widely believed that their desire for domesticity would manifest itself in lust for their wealthy male employers. There was widespread moral outrage upon the release of the ultimate governess novel, Jane Eyre. Not only did it present the governess as a subject of desire in her own right, but it also depicted a romance that crossed class lines. (Ruth Brandon's book 'Governess: The Lives and Times of the Real Jane Eyres' is a very useful resource if you have a particularly strong governess fetish.) Since then, the governess has appeared over and over again in novels and films. From the hapless Deborah Kerr as Anna Leownowens in 'The King and I' to the classic Julie Andrews character in 'The Sound of Music.' The governess is now a very strong romantic thread in the very fabric of our culture. As a fantasy figure, they run the gamut of character alignments and so are suitable for a huge range of scenarios. Maria treated the Von Trapp children like angels and has become a beloved figure in the pantheon of film history while other more sinister examples have become the epitome of discipline and corporal punishment.

Each of these characters can be incorporated into a fabulous sexual fantasy involving plenty of lascivious role playing and erotic fulfilment. The role of teenage babysitter is especially potent in that it suggests a forbidden fruit for older men. This is especially effective if their garments are cut just low enough to remind you of their womanhood, but high enough to leave plenty to the imagination. Some males will want to play the role of an older seducer, the man of the household sharing his considerable experience and expertise with the young lady. Others will want to be tempted by a brazen young Jezebel who cannot keep her passions under control. My advice is that you try experimenting with a number of combinations to see which works out most successfully. Some men might even prefer to take the role of the young ward. The tumescent teenage boy losing his virginity to an older sexy babysitter is a fantasy that many men will undoubtedly appreciate. Each of these scenarios offers endless scope for dominance and punishment for those who like their fantasies to be a little more physical. There is also the possibility of the evil babysitters dominating and humiliating her young hapless charge.

For those who wish to add a little historical re-enactment to their fantasies, baby sitting need not always be set in a contemporary milieu. Even the earliest babysitters were accused of flirting with men on street corners while the babies toddled out under the wheels of horseless carriages. If you enjoy the idea of costume play then this is perfect for the introduction of Victorian frock coats and a tightly laced bodice or two. With the governess character this can be taken to even greater heights, with costume possibilities stretching back through Edwardian and Georgian times.

The motherly ways of nannies can can also inspire a longing for 'hate sex.' While it impossible to go back and dominate the women who disciplined you as a child (teachers, bosses, mothers), you can transpose the feelings onto this lady who currently does the same thing to kids. After all, Freud says that every man suffers to some extent from the Oedipus Complex. Along those same lines of thought, crushes on hot teachers and babysitters can finally be fulfilled.

Bedtime suddenly takes on an entirely new meaning with these characters. Clothing choices are extensive but not completely necessary. In many cases an exotic accent can be much more effective than even the most elaborate costume. An au-pair can come alive with a French, Italian or even an East European accent, depending upon your personal preference. Some women might relish the opportunity to play the role of highly educated governess with a suitably 'hay clarss' accent and tone of voice. This is especially true if your partner has grown up on Jane Austin classics rather than TV soaps and endless chat shows. The naughty boy being caught by a baby sitter offers endless opportunities.

6. Back To School

Many fantasies go all the way back to our school days, as this was the time when became aware of the opposite sex for the very first time. Many a man's first attraction to girls were those in uniforms, because that is what they were surrounded by at the time. Men are and always have been very visually stimulated. When all the boys were in the throes of puberty, plaid skirts were all they saw. So even later in life, it is reminiscent of that adolescent attraction. This is very similar to the way in which most guys still think the celebrity who was popular when they were in high school is super hot, even if she is completely unknown nowadays. Catholic school girl fantasies are not restricted to one religion. Anglicans and Japanese often have exactly the same fetishes.

I did not realise the attraction of schoolgirls until my own girl started wearing pigtails when we went out. I was never aware of their power before she came along but she would give me lascivious looks while subtly playing with them all night long. Dinner was usually devoured with extreme haste or the activity cut super short so that we can get home and into the bedroom as fast as possible.

The teacher/student scenario is a classic that you can breathe new life into each and every time you play. If your girl is now an adult who wore a uniform at school, ask her if she can use it again for fantasy purposes. If she agrees then it will blow your mind for sure. If she does not still have her uniform, then it is always fun to put together a new sexy ensemble. Most teenage girls could not wait to discard the plaid skirt and starched shirt after school, but now, as a woman, it is not always so easy to find such man-fantasy relics. Of course, you can always hi-jack your niece's uniform, or order a cheap and overpriced costume online. For those of you with some teenage rebellion and lingering shock-value, the sheer volume of trashy school girl costumes available on the Internet indicate that this is a very popular role-play theme. Good costumes can really bring this one to life. For the female student, consider the following: plaid skirt or kilt, knee socks, white button-down shirt, a neck tie in coordinating colours, a coordinating cardigan, simple Mary Jane style shoes and fresh and clean underwear, such as a white cotton bra and panty set. Add to the effect with a book bag, glasses and bubble gum.

These days the Japanese Sailor Moon type sexy-school-girl is another popular alternative. If the student is relatively "innocent" go for a neat and clean look – pig tails or a crisp pony tail, fresh, natural make-up, subtle lip gloss. Of course, you can always go completely over-the-top if your student is a "bad girl" – heavy eyeliner, dark lipstick and over-styled hair.

Go shopping at your local mall. Depending on the season, you can walk away with a hot school girl costume that costs as little as $30. Begin your search in the junior section of a department store. You are looking for the classic plaid skirt. It does not matter what the trend or latest fad may be; Juniors always keep these bad boys in stock. Look for one that is short and has red in it. Once that is found, look for a simple, white cotton button up shirt. Juniors clothing designers assume the pre-teens parading their wears are no larger than an A-cup, which is exactly what you want! You are looking for a shirt that fits your waist and arms, not your breasts. Ideally, you should be able to button it up to the bottom of your bra. Finding this piece of the costume is the hardest part. Not only do you have to find something that fits (following the above stated guidelines), but you must also find a plain white shirt among a sea of glitz, glam, and Goth. Once the two staple pieces are found, you can move to the fun stuff. Department stores always have lingerie on sale. You are not searching for the Miracle Bra or one that meets your every breast needs. You are simply looking for a gaudy red pusher-upper and there is usually one on clearance or for very little. Next, you want to find some white boy shorts. Thankfully, they are the hot item at the moment. Depending on your man, you can go a step further and get character underwear such as Care Bears, Hello Kitty, or Winnie the Pooh. If you have not already figured it out by now, the bra should be worn under the partially unbuttoned top. Make sure as much of you as possible is spilling out! Do your make-up as conservative or wild as you think your man would like.

The last purchases are shoes and accessories. Perhaps you already have a pair of loafers with heels at home. If not, go to a cheap shoe store and grab the plainest pair they have. Any teeny bopper boutique can fix you up with colourful scrunches for your pigtails and dangly heart earrings.

Apart from clothes, the back to school fantasy allows for lots of interesting props. If you can, clear some space and set up a couple of desks and chairs, one for the teacher and one for the student. If you can make room for a black board, chalk and an eraser, then even better. Wooden rulers make for wonderful spanking implements, neck ties make great bondage gear, and a shiny apple is always useful as a ball gag substitute.

Ladies, remember to ask yourself, "does he want a good or bad girl?" Every man secretly longs for the virginal school girl, clad in Britney Spears-esque pigtails and uniform. Surprise your man tonight with your own version of the Teacher's Pet! If you want to play the good-girl-gone-bad role then add a few extras to your school bag. These might include cigarettes, a mini vibrator, some lube and a small flask or soda bottle filled with alcohol.

The atmosphere will be even more convincing if the teacher also has a costume. This could be along the lines of a button-down shirt (plaid perhaps), a corduroy sports jacket with elbow patches, slacks, a tie and serious looking glasses. Consider some stubble or facial hair but if clean shaven, why not look for some classic cologne such as Old Spice, Brut or Hai Karate. This will really bring back those schooldays in vivid technicolour.

Setting the Scene

Most men go directly for the bedroom to change their clothes after work. If that is the case gather a few old old textbooks (if you do not have any, go to the library - they have plenty) and knock on the door to the room he is in. Do not forget to have a lollipop in your mouth.

Ask, "Excuse me, Mr. _____, I was wondering if you had some time to help me with this homework?" It should take him a few seconds to gain composure enough to speak.

If he is into the scene and does not take you immediately, continue to play in role. Move a chair across from him and sit, legs spread and ankles crossed. Let him have a peak of what is to come. Make sure there is lots of sucking and licking on your sucker. Tell him it is hot in his office and ask if you can take off your sweater. Once that is off, the sex kitten comes out. Slowly straddle him and tell him he looks hot as well. Begin removing clothing very slowly making sure to remember to ask permission with each piece. For example, "You look really hot, Mr. _____. Do you mind if I take your tie off?" Once he is down to pants or underwear ask him if he would like to touch you. This is a good time to stop using his real family name and start calling him Mr. Big Dick instead. When he gets a little too frisky, stop him, and tell him that you have never been with anyone before. It is now time to tease and make the very most of the scenario that you have worked so hard to set up. Embarrassingly admit that you masturbate thinking of him. Ask him if he would like to watch you. Touch yourself delicately. After a few minutes, tell him that you have always fantasized about him touching you 'down there'. Continue to play it out in role as long as you can. Guaranteed, it will be a homework session neither one of you will ever forget! Expect tsunami like tidal waves of the lust that will be driving him nuts.

If you want to add more background then that is also quite easy. Think about the following questions. How have teacher and student ended up alone together? Is your student the only student in detention that day? Did the student stay after class to clean the black board brushes? Find a space in your home that you can easily transform into an imaginary classroom. Some great possibilities include an office with a desk, or a dining room with a large table. With a little imagination, these rooms can become the teacher's office or the school library.

Decide who is going to seduce whom before creating this scenario. Teacher/student role-play is hot no matter who initiates, and the power play can go back and forth. Regardless of who is taking the lead, decide that this is the first sexual encounter between these two characters. This will guarantee maximum sexual tension. Consider how each of your characters feels about the scenario. Is your student happy or annoyed to be in class/at school after hours? Does your teacher feel annoyed at having to stay with a student, or are they eager for the opportunity? The student can play oblivious to the teacher's advances at first, forcing the teacher to be truly brazen in their seduction. This works well too if the teacher feigns ignorance in the face of the student's come-on.

If you are the female student, consider sitting at your 'desk' with your knees apart just far enough to let your teacher catch a glimpse up your skirt, and act as though you have no idea you are flashing teach (or act like you know exactly what you are doing if it suits your character).

As teacher, if this is a detention scenario, think of some clever punishments for your naughty student. Perhaps they have to dust and polish your desk while you are sitting at it. Maybe they will have to shine your shoes, or spend some time on their knees filing some papers for you. You might be an old school disciplinarian and decide to hand out some corporal punishment by way of a sound spanking. The student may have some embarrassing/compromising contraband in their school bag that their teacher discovers and makes them use either solo or together for both to enjoy. Some women fantasize about receiving great oral sex from her man. She can have this played out by being the naughty school girl who is taught a 'lesson' about her body by her teacher. It is a common fantasy to get railed by a married college professor after class. This often entails being picked up and thrown across his desk, or perhaps roughly bent over it. It means papers and pencils to go flying everywhere and clothes literally being ripped off.

On other occasions, it is fun to let the tension build slowly. This can be done long before the action takes place. When discussing the fantasy with your boyfriend, do not just ask him straight out if he likes school girls. In this day and age with its strict climate of political correctness he might deny the fact completely. A much better approach is to tell him how you have been imagining that you are a naughty schoolgirl about to be spanked by a handsome male teacher...and when you look into his face, you always see the face of your partner.

Try preparing a course syllabus for the class, complete course name, date and name of instructor. Set up a start time and lay out the course requirements. For example, 'Academic standards are strictly enforced. Students must perform all assignments correctly and on time.' Refer specifically to course discipline, stating in writing that 'Students who fail to maintain these academic standards are liable to an over-the-knee spanking administered by the instructor.' Extracurricular activities are obviously encouraged.

Once you begin your scintillating little game, you will need to improvise. Too much planning can lose the erotic tension that is supposed to build up during the play itself, spoiling it all. Therefore I do not want to write a complete script for you to act out but here are a few ideas just to get you started.

Have the teacher meet the student outside the class room and consult his watch. In a stern tone admonish the student for being late to class. The student will reply dreamily with a nervous giggle.

"Well, in school, time in important. It would be well to remember that, young lady. Now go in the classroom; I'll be there presently."

The student saunters provocatively into the room, walking away with a exaggerated sway to her hips, the hem of her short skirt bobbing up and down precariously, flaunting herself in a very naughty fashion.

As the teacher, wait until she is inside the room and out of sight. In fact, give her a few additional minutes.

As the student, realise that instead of sitting in the desk, sitting on the floor can present a very seductive vision. Sitting up against one of the walls with your knees drawn up and her arms nonchalantly wrapped around them will allow the entire undersides of your thighs to be exposed. The view this position gives of your panties will be intoxicating - the panty bottoms coming upward from the floor and forming a delicate white triangle as they disappeared between your legs. This will cause any teacher's mouth to go dry, as you turn up your eyes innocently to him, as he is stood dumbstruck in the doorway.

As a teacher, it is appropriate to assume a scolding tone: "Miss ___, please take your proper seat. That is not a very lady-like position, and we have a class to start!" Begin the lecture with something completely non-sexual such as Newton's second law of motion, the law gives the relationship between force and acceleration and the equation F=ma. Look for that dreamy, spacey look and start to put on the pressure. Try to remember to address your student with a formal 'Miss' style.

"You are not paying attention. You are not taking any notes. You look like your mind is somewhere off in the netherworld and definitely NOT on physics."

Ignore her expression of sweet innocence. Ratchet things up when she brightly insists "Oh, I'm paying attention."

Continue in a angry tone. "No, you are not! How do you expect to pass this course?"

"Well...I..."

"You did not hand in your last assignment. Do you have today's assignment?"

By now she should be genuinely embarrassed. "No, Sir."

"I think you have a poor attitude toward your school work."

Now she will begin to look worried. "Oh, no, Sir, I work hard. Really I do."

"You know that is not true," you say sternly. "I think today I need to teach you a lesson of a different kind. You need to be punished for your attitude and for not working up to your potential in this course."

This should make her positively alarmed. "No, please. Give me another chance. I promise I'll do better."

"No, you should have thought of these consequences before you neglected your school work. I am now forced to administer a spanking. It's for your own good."

Watch the colour drain from her face, and listen for a hint of panic in her voice. "Please, not that. I'll work a lot harder. Give me another chance...please?"

"My decision is final. Now up with you. Go over and stand in that corner. You are to stand there until I call for you. While you are there, you are to think about the spanking you are going to receive. I also want you to think about why you must be spanked. When I ask, you are to tell me exactly why you deserve this spanking."

This is the time when most people act too quickly. It is much better to let the tension build of its own accord. While clad in her scanty schoolgirl outfit, give her time to think about what was going to happen to her - getting spanked, being placed over your knee, the loss of control, the exposure - all these thoughts and feelings are an important psychological component to make her fantasy real. Let her thoughts and imagination percolate. Wait a full five minutes. As the uncertain time lingers on, watch as she fidgets with her skirt more and more.

Walk back into the room, and make the following rather formal announcement: "Miss ___, please follow me to my office." Take her by the hand and lead her into the living room where you have placed a dining room chair in the middle of the room. Walk hand-in-hand and feel her gripping you hand tightly. This will give you a good idea of how excited she is. This physical contact is an important prelude to her spanking, but it will also have an effect on you. Your hand will be tingling at her touch and your heart will start to beat faster and faster.

Do not lead her all the way to the chair but stop about six feet from it. At this stage she will be begging your forgiveness in a small, trembling voice.

"Please Sir, I...I'm sorry...please..."

"No, say nothing more. I told you what I would be asking you." Release her hand and have her stand facing you. "Now tell me, young lady, why you are going to be spanked?"

In a mere whisper she will answer, "Because I have not been doing my school work properly."

"That is the main reason," you must responded sternly. "You have also been most unladylike in your manner. Now walk over to that chair, bend over, and hold the chair with both hands. Do not remove your hands from the chair while I administer your spanking or I shall have to give you a longer spanking."

Continue the dialogue all the way.

"I am now going to lift your skirt and begin your spanking." Take the hem of her skirt in your hand, and slowly raise it over her back.

By now everybody's passions will be running wild, and your hearts will be beating a mile a minute, but it is time to begin. Once she is warmed up, change the tempo a little.

"No, Miss ___, this will not do. Your misbehaviour has been blatant, more than just neglecting your studies. You need an over-the-knee spanking."

Look for a mortified expression. "No, Sir, please, not that...not that way."

"You have been a very naughty girl, and your spanking must be over the knee. Perhaps after that bottom of yours is soundly spanked, it will not sway so provocatively as you walk. Perhaps also your skirts will not be quite so short and...revealing. Yes, I must administer your spanking over my knee. It is for your own good. Now you think about that, young lady. Wait here for me. Look at that chair and seriously ponder what is going to happen to you in it when I return. Do not sit down."

Leave her to simmer, while you go to the bedroom, and come back with a pillow. The more misdirection you use, the more convincing the fantasy will feel.

Sit down on the chair, and place the pillow across your lap. This will make it more comfortable for her and raise her bottom up a bit higher, giving her the ability to squirm more easily.

Dialogue will increase the erotic nature of your actions. This is an important factor in maximizing the sexual tension in her fantasy.

Take special and deliberate care to give her entire body an appreciative, male scan from her head to toe, nodding your head with evident satisfaction.

"Now, Miss _____, I am going to begin your spanking. Your voluptuous bottom is going to feel a stinging sensation."

After five or six spanks stop and begin rubbing her bottom gently with your full hand. Describe what you feel and it will have a profound effect on her. "You have a very shapely and youthful figure," as you caress her thighs. "It's a very sensual experience to run my hands over your soft, graceful legs."

When you resume her spanking, use an irregular rhythm so that she can not predict when the next stroke will fall. This will add to her tension. Feel conscious of spanking her slowly, deliberately, savouring each individual spank on that round, feminine behind. Make sure that she feels strong hands holding her firmly in place as you spank her.

Continue the erotic dialogue. "It is very pleasant to spank you. With you held firmly in place over my knee, your helpless though delectable panty-covered bottom presents a very erotic target. But I think we need to do one more thing. Yes, I think for a final lesson, you must be spanked on your bare bottom."

This should bring immediate pleading.

"Oooh, no, Sir. Not without my panties...that's...that's...oh, that's too embarrassing. I've learned my lesson. I'll study a lot harder, I'll act more modest...please, not on my bare bottom..."

"Do not contradict me, young lady. I know best, and this is for your own good. I am going to lower your panties and spank your bare bottom."

Pause for effect and then take the waistband of her panties and slowly lower them down to just above her knees. Put one hand on each half of her bottom, and massage and squeeze them for a few moments. Wait for her excitement to over power her trepidation. Listen to her voice. If it is marginally huskier and not as smooth as it usually is, then she is nervous and your actions are working well.

When role-playing a real spanking, the dialogue leading up to the spanking and during the spanking is a very important part of creating its erotic effect. What is said is carefully crafted to intensify her feelings of submissive surrender. The talk is stern at the beginning and becomes more erotic as the game progresses. The later stages also include explicitly sexual actions. Compliment each other as you enjoy how hot you are together. Be dirty with the compliments. We all love to hear these things, believe me.

Not everybody realises that a simple spanking also has some useful physiological effects. A woman's bottom is one of her important erogenous zones, but the nerves are deeper and require harder stimulation to trigger. A spanking supplies that stimulation. Then too, the physiological process of sexual arousal demands that before orgasm can occur, blood must be collected and kept in the primary erogenous zones. Spanking creates just such a response. The stinging of the skin in a light, playful spanking causes blood to collect in her bottom and simultaneously in the other nearby erogenous zone. Thus spanking accomplishes 'mechanically' what caresses and kisses do psychologically.

Imagine for a moment that you have misbehaved and need to be spanked. You walk over to where he is sitting on the couch and reluctantly lie face down across his lap. He lifts your skirt and pulls your panties down. You feel ashamed and humiliated while he spanks you hard over and over. As you get spanked you can feel his erection bulging through his pants and in turn you start to get wet. You begin to grind your hips into his erection which only makes him angrier. He hits you harder until it starts to feel almost too good. His blows start to gravitate from your butt cheeks closer to where your vagina. He roughly sticks a finger inside you, causing you to let out a long moan. This is unexpected but it feels wonderful. You grind into his lap harder, his bulge is rock hard now. He is fingering you roughly and you are so wet. "Fuck me" you whisper and he throws you off his lap and then bends you over the couch.

Everybody knows the I-want-an-'A'-professor scenario, where the luscious young coed attempts to brown-nose the professor, flatter him, and make him feel smart and wise. Even once she is in his bed with him she will continue these obvious, transparent manoeuvres. She might even think that he is a jerk, but is willing to play this game to get what she wants. Of course, your own partner has presumably never done this sort of thing, but may know of girls who have. They may have received grades better than hers in the same courses and it is likely that she would like to see such conniving little bitches get their come-uppance. This perspective can add an interesting new perspective to the regular schoolgirl fantasy.

Have her make an appointment to see the professor concerning her classroom performance. She discusses her work with him in the course. She makes it clear to him how desperately she needs a good grade. She must maintain a certain average to be eligible for a prestigious university program. He tells her to work hard, of course, to study, etc. She crosses and uncrosses her legs, and leans forward, etc. She invites, without speaking, him to place his hand on her body. She looks at him piteously. She is all innocence. She needs an 'A' so desperately. Is there no way she can obtain this grade? "I am willing to do anything, anything!" she tells him. His hand touches her body. "Oh, Sir!" He removes hand. She leans forward again. "Yes," she whispers, "anything." Now she is crying. To comfort her, he places his arms about her shoulders. She looks up, helpless, tears in her eyes. Her lips are parted. "You excite me," she tells him. His hand strokes her waist, on the side. "Does this excite you?" he asks. "Yes," she whispers, "yes!"

Maybe he takes her roughly on his desk or perhaps on the couch in his office. It is at this point it becomes even more delicious to the female. She is now the student pretending to herself that "she is putting one over on him." But, slowly, it becomes evident to her that, given the Professor's harsh commands and instructions to her, that she has a great deal more than she bargained for. She is not going to be permitted to lie down and bounce. He, carefully and methodically, puts her through an incredible set of paces. Never had she expected anything like this. She is forced, in exacting and delicious detail to perform, and perform superbly. When she is finished she has been completely and humiliatingly had.

She is then told to put on her clothes and leave.

"What about my grade?"

She is then informed that she should work hard, and study, and so on

Now is the time to feign the rage, indignation and humiliation that such a girl would feel.

At this point the "professor" may again, if he wishes, take her once more in his arms and caress her into a fiercely resented ecstasy.

Is this not what such girls really deserve? Surely much more than "A's."

This is a kind of vengeance fantasy against women who use their sex to advance themselves. Most women despise such women. This gives her an opportunity, in imagination, to revenge herself on such unfairly competing harlots.

For many role playing can add a very special kind of romantic intimacy, making the passion more intense and erotic. An element of fantasy is important if a sex life is to endure. Experts say that if you never have any fantasies, you can easily find yourself falling into a rut and getting bored with sex. It is a really romantic way to add more excitement to lovemaking.

An alternative that I like to play is where I take the role of school janitor, and she plays class monitor or even school prefect. Sometimes I will catch her in the basement smoking a joint, a misdemeanour that could easily have her expelled from school. It is then up to her to persuade me that I should not report her to the headmistress. It is only later that I transform from mild mannered janitor into a demanding sexual sadist, ensuring that she receives a punishment from me far worse than could have ever dreamed of receiving from the headmistress. The scenario often ends like a basement S&M scene from a Tarrantino movie.

On other occasions, I take on the role of the Max Cady character as played by Robert De Niro in the remake of Cape Fear. Robert De Niro poses as the new drama teacher seducing a very young looking Juliette Lewis, playing the character of Danielle Bowden. Following the lead of this deranged maniac allows me to go completely off the handle, something which turns on my partner immensely.

In fantasies such as these, the relationship played out is one in which one character has authority and control over the other. This is always very exciting for both parties. If the roles can be twisted even further then the effects are usually intensified. The erotic effect is greatly increased by role playing, and really acting them out together. This is what really heightens sexual tension and anticipation.

Remember that the the female need not always take the role of the student. Sometimes it is fun to reverse the roles completely and play the role of a naughty boarding school student as a male submissive. In this variant on the classic "naughty Catholic schoolgirl," this fantasy scenario features a male boarding school student who is caught by the headmistress doing something unspeakable—maybe masturbating, or perhaps reading a dirty magazine. The stern headmistress must then discipline the schoolboy. Spankings and other corporeal punishment is a good place to start; or perhaps he will be stripped and made to stand in the corner, or be stripped and have his genitals bound, or be forced to beg the headmistress or headmaster for permission. In any event, if he becomes aroused during the punishment, then he will be in much more serious trouble...which may include more direct and painful punishment.

Decide in advance if your student is a good boy or a bad boy – clean cut and clean-shaven works well for good boy. Messy or over-styled hair and stubble for bad boy. Twill pants in a dark colour, collared shirt or button down in white, a tie, dark shoes and white boxer briefs

Pay plenty of attention to the teacher's uniform. Start with a really tight button down shirt showing off the maximum amount of cleavage possible. The skirt should be tight and form fitting. The shorter the better. Put some red lipstick on and put your hair up. High heels, lacy lingerie and a string of pearls will add greatly to the effect. Lick your lips a lot, stroke a ruler, and threaten him with detention. Tell him his grades are slipping and he needs to stay after class for extra credit. If you are wearing glasses, take them off when you get down to business, and consider letting your hair down too.

Erotic role play, when two people play roles and act out their fantasies, is a terrific way to add spice and exciting variation to your usual sexual routines. Role play, because you tap into your shared fantasies, takes an already-great sex life and makes it extraordinary, gives it new dimension, and adds playfulness - or intensity - to your intimacy.

7. BLACKMAIL

Now that we live in the digital age, incriminating photos and home made sex tapes are a little passé. I would instead suggest a common internet based background to use a background story.

The victim has been engaged in a steamy online affair with an anonymous lover that they met on the web. At first they exchanged revealing photos, shots that became increasingly explicit as time went on. The relationship culminated in a mutual satisfaction session on Skype that was being recorded at the other end. The result is an highly embarrassing episode that could be sent to the victims friends and family if they do not meet the demands of their blackmailer. If you want, you can play out of all this build up or you can head straight to the direct contact. Once you are there in person you can use this as leverage to have them performing all kinds of degrading sex acts.

Of course, this is just one scenario in which the victim can have a secret past - some dark, shameful thing he or she has done, which his or her spouse absolutely, positively must never learn about. One day, a person out of this dark past shows up on the submissive's doorstep, with incriminating evidence in hand, threatening to expose their secret. Desperate, they try to bribe the blackmailer with sexual favors, trading sex for the secrecy. The blackmailer may make any demands on the submissive's body; the submissive is forced to comply, or be exposed.

The role of the woman here is a demanding one, calling for a range of responses and reactions. In this fantasy, as in almost all of these fantasies, the pleasures are multiplied in proportion to the capacity of the players to literally "become the characters involved," to feel as they feel, and react as they would react. Remember that you are, in these fantasies, another person, to whom these things, in their full reality, are in fact occurring. Try to fully imagine your responses and miseries, for example, to find yourself in a terrifying blackmail situation. Maybe you fear and hate your tormentor but you must serve them with perfection. And, too, perhaps much to your shame and horror, time and time again, you find yourself, as you lie in the arms of these men, trying to resist them, clutching at them and yielding to their touch, responding to them, to their scornful amusement, with mad, helpless orgasms. You are experiencing endless sexual ecstasy and yet you are miserable. You cannot help it that a man's touch, for some reason, crazes you with sexual passion.

Other than blackmail, there are always other desperate situations that can be role-played. Anybody that has seen the movie, Grifters will recall the steamy scene where Annette Benning seduces the landlord rather than pay her rent. In this case, maybe you are the landlord and your tenant realises that she simply cannot afford to pay her rent this month.

8. BLINDFOLDED LOVERS

In many of these fantasy situations I have discussed introducing as many sensual stimuli as possible, tactile, visual, olfactory, etc. This particular game instead concentrates on non-visual stimuli. The reason for this is to sharpen the many other senses that we are able to experience. These might include the urgent thumping of a heartbeat, the sound of heavy breathing, the moving of bodies, the texture of surfaces, pheremonal odours and exotic tastes. It only takes one or two experiences of making love in this fashion for your awarenesses become broadened and deepened. A woman's body, for example, with its delicate, sensuous curves, its subtle sweetness to the touch of the tongue, its sounds, as it moves and breathes, vital with life and passion, its wet, hot odours of sexual heat, is an amazing creation. It can be thrilling, for example, to know the feel and sound of her body in orgasm, to hear her breathing, to hear her cries and moans, to feel her body hot and quaking, your hands on her, to sense the writhing of her legs, the helplessness of her marvellous sexual surrender. Just be careful you do not make her squirt so bad that you both slip over and crack open your skulls. This game constitutes, in effect, an intimate course in woman appreciation. From the woman's point of view, too, of course, unable to see the man, she can become, too, undistracted by visual stimuli, much more aware of additional dimensions of sensuality.

If you wish, this can be placed in the context of a much larger fantasy. Perhaps you are slaves being mated, and the owners do not permit you the dignity of seeing each other; perhaps they do not wish complications which might arise from your seeing your mate, such as, perhaps, later recognizing one another, and maybe, falling in love. Perhaps the slave masters do not permit the slaves to converse with each other. In order to degrade the slaves, the relationship is reduced to that of a stud male and a breeder female.

A man and a woman are fastened together. Body closeness builds sexual desire. If both of you are right handed, the right hand of the girl is handcuffed to the left hand of the man. This restraint on her right hand makes her feel more vulnerable; and, of course, it leaves your right hand dangerously free.

Being fastened to a woman is a very sexy experience. If a husband and wife seem to be "growing apart," this is a good way to remind him of her essential and desirable femaleness. For best results the couple must be fastened together for some hours before. The wait builds sexual tension and desire. Handcuffs are a little overkill here. Cord or rope connecting the two wrists together is also effective, and, too, permits more freedom. If the hands are separated by some two feet, it will be easier for them to complete the regular household chores together, etc. A light chain, fastened with small padlocks is very good for this purpose. The chain should not be more than some two feet in length. Chain is very sexy, probably because of the connotations of bondage and slavery. You cannot easily free yourself from a chain; thus, subconsciously, you feel more a helpless prisoner; this can be sexually stimulating, particularly to the weaker partner who find themselves in a sexual situation without escape. Once in bed, for greater freedom, only the two ankles need be fastened together. Perhaps she is a captured criminal, or spy, and he is an apprehending officer, who has unusual plans for her, or another spy, who will take her to some secret place where she can be suitably interrogated, emptied of information, and then kept as a sex slave, etc. It is very arousing to be fastened to a woman. It is not simply that there is a sweet, enforced closeness, but you are very conscious of her movements; and, of course, vice-versa. The link causes you to sense her much more deeply.

We tend, incidentally, to have certain proximity distances which are observed in our culture. Normally these are violated only in emotionally heightened situations, mainly combat or love. If a couple is fastened within the borders of the other's space, this generates, psychologically and mechanically, a very intimate and overwhelming awareness of one another. It is then very hard for a man and a woman to become so intimately and overwhelmingly aware of one another, without becoming acutely conscious of the possibility and desirability of, the other as a sexual partner.

Try also the fantasy of simulating sex with a stranger. Blindfold him and lead him into a dark room, telling him to wait there. You might want to tie up his hands, although that is not completely necessary as long as he obeys you. You then tell him to wait for someone else to come in. Leave him for a few minutes and then come back in quietly and pretend to be a stranger. Now you can do whatever you want to him, but the important word here is slowly. The longer you take turning him on, the more he will want you. And remember, by stopping him seeing he has to rely on his other senses more, so talk to him in whispers and make as many sexy noises as you can when you start to touch him.

9. BOUND CAPTIVE

Few lovers know how use their hands well in making love. The hands are just as important as the lips, tongue and teeth in sexually stimulating the partner. In this fantasy, the lovers are forced to rely heavily on these often neglected, even ignored instruments of love.

One partner is forced to make love, with their hands tied behind their back. She, for example, is the bound captive of the great Kublai Khan, the living plunder of his latest battle campaign. Her village has been torched, the men enslaved and now she is destined to be slain unless she can make the most superb and impressive love to him. But her hands are bound! She feels helpless and is thrown into confusion. She realizes that she must try to please him, and do it exquisitely well, without the use of her hands. Otherwise she will be executed. She crawls into his bed, hands bound, as he waits. With every part of her body, her breasts, her feet, her thighs, her beautiful lips and teeth and tongue she addresses herself to his pleasure. After trying this fantasy once or twice the woman will have learned the fantastic potentialities of her body in making love.

After she has learned to do this well you can imagine how marvellous she will be when she has the use of her hands as well. This same fantasy, of course, like many, or most, of these fantasies can be used turnabout, with the male in the position of submission. Indeed, women may enjoy this when the male is bound. Having love made to them by a bound male can enhance their sense of power.

There are a great many scenarios that can be created for this simple activity. Where I live, Mongolian tribesman marauding their way across the steppe is especially appropriate but you can try any number of alternative back stories. The publicly enslaved princess is particularity effective for western women in that it creates a stark contrast between their prior success and their imminent helplessness. This makes a very stimulating transition. Imagine that there has been a long and bloody conflict. The losers were commanded by a proud and beautiful queen, who is now a prisoner of the conquerors. If you prefer she could be a general's daughter or a royal princess. She could be a consul's wife or a defeated warlord's concubine. The choices are only limited by your imagination. In regal garments, chained to the chariot of her conqueror, an emperor or general, walking behind it, the vanquished female of noble blood is paraded through the streets, exhibited as booty of his triumph. At the climax of his triumph they are, in a great square, before thousands, publicly enslaved. They are stripped, branded, collared, and publicly taken. They are then led away in chains, as common slave girls.

Many women, on some level or another, wish to be proud of their bodies and their sexual responsiveness. They also wish, at some level, to be sexually had, fully and completely. It is hard to imagine a woman more had than one who is taken by force, to show publicly, before thousands, her responsiveness, one who is exhibited and owned. The 'Enslaved Queen' fantasy combines many desirable elements of female sexual fantasy. High station, pageantry, capture, bonds, exhibition, the reduction from the highest of the high to the lowest of the low, public sex, abject enslavement. The female was once the highest person in her state, uncountably rich, whose word was law. Then she fell captive. Still she was treated with graciousness and honour, great respect. But, in the square, on the high platform, all of this ends forever. There she is enslaved. She is now only an article of property, collared and branded, to be bought or sold. She is no longer to be respected. She may now be abused and treated harshly. She must now obey masters. She who was once the queen is now only the female slave of her conquerors. It might now be the general who will keep her as his personal slave. Doubtless he will well teach her the meaning of her brand and collar. Here, as in other fantasies, there are many variants. She might prefer to think of herself as staked out, in a helpless position, perhaps arched over shields, head down, legs split, to satisfy the lust of an army. If a vibrator is used, each thrill of sensation can be imagined by her as her rape by a new soldier. Once this public humiliation is complete, then the slave can be marched away to the confines of the Emperor's tent where she must act out the role of bound captive that I described at the beginning of this chapter.

Some women have far more extreme fantasies. She imagines that she has been wrongly convicted, or framed, and yet, though innocent, are condemned to the public brothel. Perhaps the individual who framed her, whom she once spurned as a lover, now visits her regularly and makes her serve him, perfectly. As she responds to him in orgasm she begs him to again propose marriage, but he merely calls her a bitch, and leaves her to her chains, behind the bars.

Imagine perhaps a bound sex slave in a large brothel being whored out to male customers. The place is like a strip club, open plan, but instead of strippers, it is filled with sex slaves. Sometimes they are blind folded. All they can hear are the cries of the women, and the men groaning and degrading and abusing them. In one especially harsh scenario she is strapped down onto a heavy leather bench. Her head hangs upside-down over the edge and is strapped in place, so men can stand and abuse her facially and grope her breasts. This enables others to similarly force themselves upon her at the other end of the bench. She is simply left there as customers come and go all day doing whatever they please to the bound helpless captive. For an even more extreme fantasy imagine that she has tried to escape the facility. As a punishment she has been made the public 'cum bucket.' The cum bucket is in the centre of the room, and should be punished by all customers. There is no charge for the cum bucket. You use her as you wish, to break her and teach her a lesson. Anything goes. It is rough and violent. This is an especially exciting fantasy for women that get off on being used for someone else's sick pleasure. The foul and filthy language used as they force themselves into her are indeed one of the biggest turn-ons.

As always, there are going to be occasions when things do not work out completely as anticipated. I would be lying if I tried to tell you otherwise. Like the time that I tied my girlfriend's hands and she proceed to try and give me a foot job. It tickled her feet so bad that she started laughing and kicked me right in the bollocks. This was the same girl with whom I have my initial soixante neuf experiments. As hyped up as 69 was, I was greatly disappointed and had to stop her after she farted in my face for the third time. Don't get me wrong, the blow-job was spectacular - I just did not think I could handle 66 more farts. The more she got into giving me head, the more she sat on my face, until my nose was literally vacuuming up the farts. You would think that this would be the one time you could hold it in no matter how hard it was. But no!

Still I am no angel on that score myself. I remember getting a blow-job in the back of my car. I was hammered and had been stuffing myself with pizza and buffalo wings all day. I was mid-blow-job with this girl I had just met and of course right then I just had the uncontrollable urge to fart. I tried so hard to hold it in but it just came out, and loud too. I was so embarrassed but the girl laughed it off and kept going. I farted twice more in short succession and just had to get out of the car and tell her I was sorry.

10. BREAKING AND ENTERING

The burglar scenario is a great fantasy for guys to spring on girls. Call your lady friend. Tell her you have heard that there are burglars in her neighbourhood, who prey on the type of young, beautiful, single woman who traipses around her apartment at 8:00 in the evening wearing sexy lingerie. They tie these women up, ransack their bedrooms, then have their wicked way with their helpless victims. They seldom even have to break in, because these women are the scatterbrained type who leave their front doors unlocked. Lay it on with a trowel. Make it abundantly clear to your lady friend that she should be lounging around her place in lingerie with the front door unlocked at 8 o'clock tonight.

Later, you go over to her place at 8, wearing a burglar costume: Black shirt, black slacks, leather gloves, a swag bag, and a mask of some kind. When you buzz, announce "Burglars!" in a friendly voice (assuming there is nobody else in the lobby.) Go up to her apartment. Open the door. Tiptoe around until you find your lady, hopefully dressed to please you. You could "chloroform" her by holding a handkerchief soaked in cheap cologne lightly over her nose and mouth for a few seconds; Or she could obligingly faint at the very sight of you. Or you can simply seize her in your strong, manly arms. The result is the same: She gets bound and gagged in her bedroom, where she must sit/lie helplessly while you go through her dresser drawers, take her costume jewellery, rummage in her purse, and generally violate her space. Then you can violate her. After you have taken everything of value, you leave her tied up and go. (Danger warning! Do not go out any doors that lock!) Just go a short distance away. Wait a few minutes. Put on a different shirt, and take off the mask. Then go back into the bedroom with a cheerful, "Here I am to protect you from the burglars -

Heavens! What happened!!" Untie her, take her in your arms, comfort her an any way she may desire. See how many ways she can show her gratitude for being rescued.

For people whose tastes are a bit spicier, you can do the same sort of scenario with less warning. Call your partner and tell her you have just seen a news report that says there is a burglar in the area. Then, dress as a burglar, and creep into the house. Catch your partner by surprise, physically overpower her, and have your way with him or her. In a reversed version, she is the burglar - black leotard, black tights, high-heeled boots and mask. She sneaks into his apartment, and begins rummaging through his things. Suddenly the lights go on – she is caught! He ties her up to hold her for the cops. She pleads with him, and offers 'anything' if he will let her go. Of course, she need not always fall into the role of the submissive. If she is the perpetrator, then there is no reason why she would not be armed and fully able to force him into submission. I think if you ask any man, most will tell you that as youngsters they had quite detailed fantasies about sexy, female cat-burglars breaking into their bedrooms late at night.

A similar setting is that of the night-watchman or security guard. The submissive has committed some infraction - perhaps trespassing on secure property while walking home late one night. The security guard confronts the offender, and takes them back into the security room, where they are subject to a humiliating strip search. The security guard explains that standard policy is for the police to be notified and the offender is to be booked for criminal trespass, but that other arrangements can be made; at this point, wishing to avoid a night in jail, the offender does whatever the security guard instructs. As a variation, the security guard is required by company policy to videotape the search, to prevent liability problems; after the guard and the trespasser reach their agreement, the guard continues to videotape the trespasser while the guard molests him or her, just to add to the humiliation.

Sometimes the burglar scenario takes quite a bit of organising. I would like to relate my own experience in helping a a friend stage a fake break and enter so that he could fulfil his girlfriends rape fantasy. Maybe this will inspire you to help out one of your friends should the need ever arise.

My friend new that I was a very dominant character, playing all kinds of sex games with my own partners. He himself was far less experienced in this area and decided to ask for my help. His new girlfriend had told him that she was fascinated by the whole rape fetish thing. She described a fantasy where an intruder breaks in, beats her boyfriend to a pulp and then brutally rapes her. My friend is far too nice and meek to ever want to try that sort of role playing so he said no and she was obviously very disappointed. He told me that he looked at him with sad puppy dog eyes, like he had cancelled Christmas at the orphanage and then given Santa a kicking while the children looked on.

He went into a lot of details saying how he would really like to make this fantasy come true for her but did not know how. Initially, I jokingly suggested that we stage a fake break-and-enter rapery; smash a pane of glass in a kiddie pool in his living room, he comes in, we yell at each other, pretend to fight, I make it to the bedroom look at her licentiously, he pulls me back through the door, we tussle again, whilst he slips on my balaclava and shoes, takes off his pyjamas to reveal the same clothes that I am wearing as he goes back in and has his way with her to her heart's delight, while I get the hell out of Dodge. We were pretty much the same build and so it would be easily believable. He looks at me as if I have just solved the Riemann hypothesis, tells me that is a brilliant idea and asks if I would really help him pull it off.

For me it was a real adventure. I love all of this role-play cosplay malarkey and was more than happy to be of assistance. Amazingly it all went off without a hitch. I will leave the more intimate details of the degree of success to you imagination, but suffice to say that it went perfectly. Of course he never said which of his friends helped him out but I have a feeling that she has guessed. I never really got on with the girl before and she began acting a little weird afterwards. She began being really nice to me and for a while I was worried that it was going to turn into "Gee, that was fun, it sure would be great to be brutally raped by TWO robbers!"

11. Capture In The Dark

This is a very simple fantasy. The room is pitch dark. You do not know the location of your partner, who is nude, somewhere in the room. You find her, capture her and take her to your bed. Then, over a period of an hour or so, you give her an exquisite ravishment, all in utter darkness.

During the capture phase, there should be a struggle. Even so, it must be clearly understood that this is to be a lovers' wrestling, in which each is concerned that the other not be injured. When she loses, they both win. There is no game, of course, if she gets smacked in the head or he gets mashed in the testicles. That would be like hitting the opposing pitcher with a baseball bat. In all love struggles, there must be delight. They are mock fights, not real combat. Each must take care to avoid hurting the other; their second job, of course, is to see that each gets as much pleasure as the other can give. If he then turns her to her back, and, a hand under the back of each knee, thrusts her back against the head of the bed or, if on a rug, against the wall, she can struggle as much as she pleases. She has nowhere to go and she is confined. If she continues to struggle her movements will merely add to your delectation. Every woman likes a hint of danger; it is like perfume to a man. She will not think less of her partner, knowing he can take her when he wants. She might even find it sexually stimulating. It does not hurt a woman's libido to understand that her lover may not be as harmless as she thought. A woman who is fantasy raped by her lover is likely to remember the event long after she has forgotten more prosaic love makings. Under normal lighting conditions visual stimulation adds much to the joy of the fantasy, as it does to most love makings. In the capture-in-the-dark fantasy, however, we have the element of the hunt, and the delight of the catch, when you apprehend her. It appeals to the hunter in you and the quarry in her. Furthermore, human beings have a fear, commonly, of the dark. In this case, the fears of being caught in the dark are a source of stimulating excitement, for you both know there is, truly, no danger. It is only a fantasy. Similarly, the darkness, concealing the lovers from one another, makes it easier to suppose and fantasize that it is a delicious stranger whom you have caught and forced to your bed. For her, it is some unknown, magnificent, mysterious male, who has captured her and will now force her to respond to the enormities of his lust.

Mechanics can vary endlessly in these fantasies. For example, the predator may or may not desire to bind his prey before he takes it to his bed, or den. He might force her to walk, or he might carry her. She could be in his arms, bound or unbound, or over his shoulder, again bound or unbound. He might speak, or or he could remain strong and silent. She may plead with him for her freedom, or be gagged taken in silence. If she is not originally nude when captured, but wears, say, stockings, panties, garter belt and brassiere, she carries with her her own bonds and gag. Stockings are excellent for binding her, one for the hands, one for the feet. Her other garments are already removed. The garter belt is discarded; the panties serve as wadding. Then, secured, she is yours. Carry her to your bed.

Once in bed, if you choose to unbind her and ungag her, you may wish to secure her there or on the floor at the foot of the bed. A length of chain, with two padlocks, fastening her by the left ankle, or the throat, to the bed, might please her. For extra effect, she is pulled by the hair to her feet and then she is walked to the bed, bent over, her hair held at your waist. This makes a woman feel very much in a man's power. She is marched around the room a few times. Now her back and the back of her legs, and her hair, will begin to hurt. Also, she is humiliated, being led about as such a captive. Then, by the hair she is thrown across the bed.

Another variant on this fantasy reverses the roles, and has the man be the victim. In this case, perhaps the woman is large, strong and fierce voodoo priestess. To his horror he finds himself overpowered, as easily as he might have overpowered an ordinary woman, and treated with the same lust and casualness that he might have inflicted on a woman in his position. Many fantasies have turnabout possibilities. Another variant here would be that she is an evil Medici Duchess who has captured him for her pleasure. In spite of the fact that he is larger and stronger than she, she handles him swiftly and efficiently. To her he is simply a clumsy victim. He fears her for he knows that, as her beauty tortures and torments him, she can do with him as she pleases. He must obey her. She, like that of a dog, is his mistress.

12. CRIME PAYS

Maybe it is the uniform. Or the handcuffs. Or maybe it is simply the power held by a police officer that makes role playing cop and criminal so spicy. The police officer fantasy seems to be pretty strongly shared by both genders. A uniform is an immediate reinforcement of authority in our minds. And that is not to mention the sexy side of breaking the law – it is taboo, and everything forbidden has an inescapable hint of the erotic. This role-play is full of sexual tension. This is where it is really good to be the bad guy! Arrest your partner, read them their rights, and have them surrender to your love! They might not stay quite so silent though, officer! Turn around, put your hands behind your back, and spread em'! Definitely make an effort to find a good cop costume for this role play. Post-Halloween clearance is a good time to stock up on items for your erotic closet. Props help, too – handcuffs are almost mandatory. When playing with handcuffs, always know where the key is! Have a spare or two on hand and keep them in your wallet or purse.

Once you are ready to explore the ins and outs of crime and punishment, begin by creating some ridiculous rules and regulations. One such 'rule' might be Attempted Seduction; another could be Aggregated Sexiness, or Possession of a Dangerous Body. Or she can wear hooker clothes, and stand on the corner of Driveway and Garage Door when he drives home. She makes him an offer, only to learn that he is a vice cop. She is placed under arrest. He makes her "spread 'em", frisks her, and ties her hands – it has been a busy night, they are out of handcuffs. This can also explain why she is tied to a chair in the squad (bed) room instead of going to lock-up. If she starts mouthing off to the arresting officer, he might even gag her. She might be sentenced to a spanking, or she might be able to bribe the officer with her body

Alternatively, you have apprehended a female suspect accused of hiding contraband on her person. It could be drugs, it could be a stolen watch, it could be an illegal weapon. A brief frisking of the handcuffed suspect does not reveal the contraband's hiding place, but the police officer is sure she is concealing it somewhere. Obviously, the next step is to perform a strip search. A very thorough strip search. After that, the body cavity probe. Soon the suspect is sure to cooperate with the investigation, one way or another – no matter where that nightstick finally ends up.

I heard of one man whose wife fantasised about them being caught dogging, that is engaging in public sex. She dreamed about being bundled naked into the back of patrol car or better still a Black Maria police van filled with officers. They were all laughing at her and humiliating her but at the same time all getting excited at seeing her without any clothes. As drove her away, leaving hubby in the car park they stopped half way to the police station, telling her that if she cooperated it would go much better for her once they get back to the station. In the fantasy, she ends up servicing all of them in the back of the van as they grope her and abuse her.

If you want to reverse the roles, then remember that a lady police officer is one tough nut to crack. She has had to be better than the boys her entire career – smarter, stricter, rougher. She knows the procedure and does things by the book. It is going to take a wily criminal indeed to get her to bend the rules. A sexy smooth-talker who clearly poses no harm, seeing as he is in handcuffs already. But if she needs to frisk him, that is fine too. Can he charm her into letting him go – or at least sweet-talk himself into her pants? Still handcuffed, if necessary – those bedposts sure come in handy for securing suspects sometimes.

For something slightly more edgy, playing prison guard and prisoner can be a heady little sex game. Fantasies of being dominated and coerced are actually quite common, and since most of us will never see the actual inside of a jail cell, playing these sorts of games is safely removed from day-to-day reality. There is good reason all those trashy 'women in prison' films are so popular.

The strip search scenario is always a good place to start. The prisoner is suspected of smuggling contraband into the jail – be it cigarettes, pornography, drugs, weapons or just the proverbial nail file in a cake. He or she has hidden it somewhere on his or her body. Clearly, it is time for a thorough strip and body cavity search. Do not forget to restrain your prisoner first.

In one very detailed fantasy, I read about a woman who wanted to be sentenced to an all-male prison to act as a sex toy for the inmates. She even went as far as saying that she had falsely accused a man of rape and was convicted of false testimony and sentenced in what she bizarrely thought was the most appropriate way. There was just one woman to every hundred men so she got a lot of use. By the time each inmate takes his turn, he would be suffering so much pent-up frustration and aggression which he would be welcome to release upon his toy. If a toy was injured she could spend time in toy hospital, but that inactive time would be added on to her sentence. In another element, each inmate would grade the sex slave on her 'performance', giving her a black mark if she was unsatisfactory. At the end of the week, anybody who had received black marks would receive public punishment in front of the whole prison. This was usually a public flogging of six strokes per black mark. If the number of strokes got beyond a certain level, the whipping would shift from the back to the more tender parts of the body. Of course, the inmates soon realised that it was fun to see the sluts punished, and start assigning the maximum black marks for every girl so that they would get the beating of their lives at the end of each week. Male prisoners who had stored up merit points for good behaviour would get to administer the whippings. As long as they had a good strong swing. For her the very best part of this fantasy was that the woman would go straight from their flogging back into the hands of the inmate, now in groups of three...

Of course, not all prison fantasies need to be so extreme, although the nature of the setting does tend to produce dark and brutal outcomes. If you want to start off with something a little softer then try the role a prisoner who is trying very, very hard to be good for the guards. Very, very good. In fact, the prisoner is willing to do anything to help the guards and maybe even earn some time off for good behaviour. He or she will snitch on other prisoners, shine shoes – whatever it takes. And if that should involve requests for sexual favours, well, what truly well-behaved prisoner would refuse? A variation in this is when the prisoner attempts to seduce an upstanding by-the-books guard. What will it take to break him or her down? Will the prisoner then threaten to blackmail the guard? What will the prisoner demand in return for his or her silence? Perhaps more sexual favours – or a return engagement, if you want to play this game again. It is all up to you two, together, to decide.

13. Delivery Services

When I was much younger, I had a part time job as a pizza delivery boy. The very first evening I had to deliver a pizza to a single woman's house. She paid for it, tipped me, and bid me farewell. It did not go at all as I had expected. What a complete waste of a pizza with extra sausage...

Despite my own disappointment, the pizza boy porn plot remains a popular theme in countless X-rated movies. Fortunately for me, I was able to act out the fantasy later in life with a very adventurous girlfriend. She called me on my mobile, pretending that I was the pizza house, ordering a twelve incher with extra spicy salami. I arrived at the apartment a few minutes later and rang the bell as usual. Keeping in character I waited at the door while she went into the bedroom to fetch some money. Silently, I closed the door and prepared to catch her by surprise. When she returned, I veered way off script and jumped her from behind. I tied her hands and feet with bungee cord and began to humiliate here, releasing all the pent up frustration that she had caused by always answering the door in her underwear and being such a tease. I told that she was a bitch and that her come uppence was here at last. She was going to get what she had always teased me for in spades. I put a large piece of tape over her mouth and despite her pleas fucked her eight ways from Sunday, in every way known to man and monkey. She later told me that it was the most exciting experience of her life.

Since then, I have not only played out my role, first as the UPS man with an express package for her but also as a handyman, here to fix her dripping taps.

On occasion I like her to be in the delivery role. There is something hopelessly erotic about room service. Maybe it is simply the decadence involved in ordering food that is delivered right to your bed. Maybe it is the sensual delights of food, combined with the equally sensual delights to be found between the sheets. Under the guise of room service she arrives at my at my door with coffee and tea service, complete with a few sweet treats for added pleasure afterwards. She feigns ignorance when I tell her that I did not order anything but she is very very persistent. She pours, arranges the cream and the sugar, and then asks me choose "Coffee, Tea or Me?"

Did you ever wish that you could order up more than just food from room service? Wouldn't it be nice if there was a delivery service for, shall we say, sexual novelties? And if the delivery boy or girl was a sweet slice of sexy, all the better. All you need to fulfil this dream is a tray, a plate and a plate cover. Only this time, instead of stashing food beneath the metal plate cover, you will stash a selection of your favourite sex toys. Knock on the hotel room door and, once you are let inside, remove the cover with a grand flourish. Explain what each sex toy arranged so tastefully on the plate is used for. Offer to demonstrate if necessary. Hands-on, of course. The cardinal rule of hotel role-play is: be nice to the staff. So spare everyone the embarrassment and do not get actual room service employees involved in your scene.

Housekeeping is not the only hotel service you may encounter – or fantasize about – during a hotel stay. Sometimes something goes wrong in your suite. The sink backs up, there is no hot water, the air conditioning will not turn on. Time to call maintenance! Maintenance workers tend to be on the blue-collar, less than talkative side. They wear coveralls that beg you to imagine what is underneath. And they have the keys to your room. In this role-play, one of you pretends to be the hapless guest and the other gets to, well, get handy. To set the scene, have the handyman carry a toolbox or bag. Of course, it can be filled with more "tools" than just wrenches and screwdrivers, if you know what we mean.

Isn't it awkward how the handyman always arrives at the least convenient moment – say, when you have started running the water and taken off all your clothes in preparation for a quick shower? Let him into the room anyway. Who knows when you will have another chance to get your pipes fixed? When he compliments you on the lovely picture you provide, have second thoughts about which pipes he should attend to first. There is always a opportunity for the lovely lady guest to seduce the innocent plumber. He is just trying to do his job, bending over to look under the sink or at a low outlet. And those pants always seem to hang a little too low. Slip a hand down his pants and give him a goose. Make sure he does not crack his head on the cabinet! If he does, maybe he will accept a kiss to make it better. A long, slow, romantic kiss, that is. Most likely, he will need a touch more TLC before he is ready to return to work – and you are willing to provide anything he needs. Anything at all.

There is one handyman scenario that has a kinky twist to it. The hotel guest has somehow found herself in a bit of a predicament. She has been preparing for her boyfriend's imminent arrival, locked herself into a pair of play handcuffs and she has now misplaced the key. She is wearing only the skimpy lingerie she donned before experimenting with her toys. Overcoming her embarrassment, she calls maintenance for assistance with her predicament. As the handyman attempts to free her from her shackles, things heat up between the pair. Maybe he manages to remove the handcuffs — and maybe they both decide to wait a little while longer before she is finally free.

14. DEMON SUMMONING

One of my own personal favourite sexual fantasies is the satanic ritual. I have always been fascinated by the dark supernatural forces and relish the opportunity to experiment with the dark arts in a sexual setting. I would like to share with you here some of my own tips and tricks for making this an extra special fantasy.

I usually play the role of evil mage and high priest, intending to summon a demon of the lower planes in exchange for my bound, naked partner using advanced magick of the ancients. Costumes and settings can range from the very simple to the highly ornate depending upon your level of interest and what you happen to have lying around the house. At the most basic level this can be some simple ties for the victim and a long robe from the master thaumaturgist. I went to the extent of having a large pentagram inside a satanic circle printed out that we could use as a floor covering. I copied the design from the classic house of Hammer horror movie, The Devil Rides Out (a great source of erotic inspiration) and had it printed out on to thick vinyl. With large candles at the cardinal points this totally transformed an ordinary room into a black magicians chamber. Place four candles north, east, south, west. They can be of any colour, although I prefer black ones, but you can have one of each corresponding colour on each quarter of the circle.

As ritual occultists and demonolators, we have to open ourselves to spiritual energy of an entity, allowing for natural, unrestricted communication, exchange of energies, sometimes merging of consciousnesses. Sex provides energy by creating a tension that is released in orgasms. According to Aleister Crowley, a magician so notorious that he was known as the Great Beast, sex was "the supreme magical power". I use an old book to take the place of an ancient grimoire with which I initiate contact with the astral realm. I then imagine that I am Alan Moore or a modern day Rasputin going into deep trance while receiving demonic energy from the Satanic Astral Temple.

Add as much ritual as possible to the event and feel free to read esoteric, unintelligible texts out loud. This will certainly add to the overall atmosphere. In the background, I was playing a looped Halloween special effects tape that I had downloaded from the internet. The sounds of thunder and lightning set the scene. Depending on my mood, I might have my sacrificial virgin standing in the centre of the circle. Sometimes I will have her lying spread-eagled while I conduct numerous satanic castings. Often this will include marking ancient hieroglyphs on her naked body, marking points of power with ancient characters and obscure pictograms. This was a trick that I learned from a Chinese performance artist but I have since seen it used in the movie Conan the Barbarian where Arnold Schwarzenegger has esoteric symbols painted onto his body in order to ward off evil spirits. This in turn was taken from an ancient Japanese play entitled 'Hoichi the Earless.' At some stage I will usually blindfold her and simulate a blood sacrifice. With her eyes covered, it is surprising how easy to fool her into thinking that the pressure of even a pen is a razor sharp dagger slicing into her flesh. I then collect the imaginary blood in a suitably evil looking bowl, but in reality this is usually just a small amount of ketchup that I have prepared earlier. I will draw obscure sigils onto her body with my fingers dipped in her 'blood.' If I take away the blindfold she will see the results and I will relish smearing the rest of the it onto her cheeks and forehead.

Detailed incantations can have an amazing effect. If you do not consider yourself a very competent linguist, then try starting with a simple Latin incantation:

Daemon, esto subjecto voluntati meae.

Ad ligandum eos pariter eos coram me.

If you are feeling more confident, the following summonation will cause the earth in surrounding vicinity to violently shake, until the demon is able to manifest in a nearest, suitable vessel.

Te invoco apro fundus inferni...

Attenrobendum eos, ad consiendrum, ad ligandum eos, potiter et solvendum, et ad, congregontum eos, coram me.

...Et ad congregandum...eos coram me.

Ad constringendum, ad ligandum eos pariter et solvendum: Et ad congregandum eos coram me.

If you prefer you can recite an Old Celtic incantation or perhaps even something in Tibetan will have the desired effect.

For the final summoning sequence, I prefer to replace the blindfold to make the effect even more dramatic. The first time that I did this, I used a large firework to mark the appearance of the demon but the noise was deafening and probably rather dangerous. These days I simply use a prepared soundtrack. I like the religious chanting from the Jerry Goldsmith's soundtrack of that classic horror film The Omen, combined with a large explosion when I temporarily turn up the volume and flash on the lights. I find that the sections from the Dog Attack are the most atmospheric parts of the CD. For anybody wearing a blindfold, the effects are very authentic. I have also used Gregorian chant as well as the guttural chanting of Tibetan Lamas, both have which have had the desired effect.

Upon the appearance of the demon I will solemnly recite the following greeting:

Welcome almighty adversary of evil. Lucifer, Your Almighty Satanic Majesty, let them praise your Great and Terrible Name, for it is Holy.

Sometimes I conjure a demon into the room where we are standing, where I quickly switch roles, instantly going from arch-mage to terrifying beast from the bowels of hell. Once the apparition is fully manifest I will offer it the victim and then pretend to leave the room, closing the door behind me. The next thing that the poor girl hears are growls coming from the far corner of the room. I don a pair of large pair of heavy work gloves and roughly manhandle her naked body, giving her the impression that she is being explored by some monstrous beast. A good way to emphasise this is through smell. In my case, I left the gloves in the bed of a friend's dog for a week or so before hand until they had a suitably animalistic scent. On other occasions, I will pretend that we have been magically transported in the depths of the abyss and will hold a conversation with his satanic majesty himself. Both have worked equally well in the past.

The abyssal plane is an interesting location in itself. The scent of incense, perfume, and oily naked bodies are thick in the air of the 69th layer of the abyss. This purgatory of perversion and licentiousness encompasses an enormous palace that stretches far and wide, far beyond the imagination. It is the home of the unholy Empress Dowager of all Succubi and Incubi. The palace is filled with demon princes and princesses of Lust, Sex, and Sodomy. Countless thousands upon thousands of succubi and incubi engrossed with every conceivable sexual act. The halls of this palace are all lined with beautiful slaves whose bodies have been painted gold, and their sexual organs made to be on display for all to see as the slaves are forced to stand in erotic positions, living statues for their demon princess. This plane gives new meaning to the idea of torturous pleasure, as the lust and desires of any slave or demon upon this plane will rarely, if ever, go satisfied for any significant period of time. Demons and monstrosities populate this plane by the thousands, but each one is always deceptively beautiful, their purpose being to seduce all intruders and slaves into their service. The pheromones that permeate this layer are such that any mortal who enters their lustful desire will become so strong that they will stop what they are doing and race to join the nearest orgy within the layer (since they are so many going on all the time, one should not be far). It is rumoured that demons and daemons from all over frequent this layer constantly when they have a chance to pursue personal pleasures.

The roles can easily be reversed and I have occasionally enjoyed being sacrificed to a malignant manifestation of the Old Order. Of course there is always the opportunity for the female to take on the role of High Priestess and transform herself into a demoness. Lucretia of the lower planes has a deadly kiss that drains all energy from a victim, leaving them doomed to serve as a pleasure slave for her, for all eternity. Her form is such that it sparks the most wanton abandon of lust and sexual desire possible in her victims minds. Her sexual pheromones are so powerful and here aura of lust and sex enough to cause any man or woman to immediately prostrate themselves naked before her.

If you too are fascinated by the occult and want to incorporate it into your sexual role playing, then I would highly recommend Donald Tyson's classic magical treatise entitled 'Sexual Alchemy' as an extensive source of inspiration. Some other good research books are The Yoga of Power by Julius Evola, Sexual Magic by Beverly Randolph Pascal translated by Robert North, Fire and Ice by S. Edred Flowers, Secrets of the German Sex Magicians by Frater U.D. and Tantrism by Benjamin Walker. Dr. Flowers and his wife Crystal run a sexual magic order dedicated to sado-shamanism called the Order of the Triskelion. Mr. North runs a sexual magic order called the New Flesh Palladium.

Once the ritual is over, then extra mileage might be made from an appearance of the Spanish Inquisition. The innocence of the female victim will be of little import to these cruel torturers.

15. DOCTORS AND NURSES

There is no question that this particular childhood game palpates and palpitates its way into adulthood, bringing new meaning to doctor-patient privilege. Taboo abounds when it comes to fetishes involving medical and hospital fantasies. Any time you engage in any role playing activities, pushing the boundaries of erotic creativity is always the name of the game, and the options for kinky quacks, sexy nurses, and the patients that love to be poked and prodded are practically endless. Doctor-patient role play is a huge turn-on for many people. Either of you can play the role of doctor, and either of you can be the patient. Part of this scenario's appeal may be the cool detachment medical professionals exhibit while you are stuck with only an oversized paper towel between you and being embarrassingly nude. Of course, in the fantasy, there is no need for the doctor to keep his or her composure.

As far as bottoms (submissive partners) are concerned, think about the real life implications of going to see a medical professional. You are usually in a vulnerable state because you are sick or injured, and all you want to do is get better. But in order to get well again, patients sometimes have to be subjected to embarrassing or, at times, even humiliating medical procedures - and they have to trust that their caretaker will do whatever is necessary to cure what ails them. And when the doc or nurse is hot, it is an extra incentive to grin and bear it. Many would contend that the desire to give in to another person so willingly, yet so unwillingly at the same time, is a mental struggle that conjures up deep primal instincts.

For the partner who chooses to be dominant in the scene, control becomes their medical speciality. Once the boundaries of play are established by each person, the doctor teases their patient to the brink of ecstasy by delivering a playful - or scolding - mix of pain and pleasure. They can promise to make the unpleasantness of an exam worth it by offering rewards for their patient's compliance, or threaten a more extensive investigation if they do not fully submit. Keep in mind that the dominant does not necessarily have to inflict pain for this fantasy to be enjoyed; the patient can simply be kept in a state of not knowing what will happen next in order to heighten sexual arousal, or they can be nurtured back to health through sexual favours.

Most of us have played variations on this game at some time in our life, usually as curious five-year-olds. And we knew back then it was naughty, which is why it still holds a thrill now that we are adults. Here is the low down on how to put the ER into erotic.

My own version of the fantasy starts with my favourite nurse coming in to change my dressing a few days after the operation. She is tall, has the most gorgeous hair and a beautiful figure. I have been eyeing her for some days and get a hard-on just thinking about her. On this particular day she comes into my private room. After closing the curtains to make the place completely private, she pulls down the bedclothes and says she wants to look at my wound to see if it is healing properly. Slowly she opens my pyjamas and pulls them down to reveal my groin. The smell of her body, the way her hair glistens in the sunlight and the presence of her so close and yet so far makes me feel extremely horny. She starts to inspect the wound and as she does so, I begin to stir. I pretend not to notice because I am so embarrassed, but it is all too obvious what is happening.

As she finishes replacing the dressing, she 'accidentally' brushes her hand against my penis, stirring me into action even more.

"I think we'd better check that this still works all right after the operation," she says, taking my penis into her hand and massaging it to produce an enormous erection.

"Seems perfectly OK to me," she whispers as she sees the effect she is having.

Then without more ado she bends down and slips it into her mouth. I am flabbergasted, but delighted. She then fellates me as expertly as I imagine any woman could and within seconds I am panting and ready to come. "Hold on," she murmurs, after taking my red, throbbing prick out of her mouth, and goes over to the door and locks it.

Before I know what is happening, she raises the skirt of her uniform and kneels on the bed astride me. I lift up the starched material to see that she is wearing black stockings with lacy tops and nothing else. "The sexy bitch," I think to myself, " she came here ready to fuck me. I'll show her."

Being careful not to disturb my wound, she lowers herself on to me and moans with pleasure as its swollen head stretches her wide. I am virtually immobile because I am lying down and because frankly, I am scared to death to do too much in case I burst my stitches.

"This should take the pressure off your groin and let the wound heal," she whispers as she moves rhythmically up and down.

I reach under her starched white apron and fondle her breasts. She caresses herself.

Just at that moment someone knocks on the door. It is the head nurse wanting to come in.

"We won't be a moment," my nurse calls out in a stifled voice and, within seconds, she shudders with her orgasm and I shoot inside. Without saying a word she gets off me, covers me up, straightens her uniform and leaves the room, pausing only to give me a backward glance and a satisfied smile that I shall remember for the rest of my life.

You do not actually need much equipment to play out hospital fantasies. Pack lots of latex gloves, plus any other medical equipment you might have to add to the ambience. Who has not raided their doctor's drawers when they were out of the exam room? A lite kit containing kinky medical gadgets can be put together fairly easily by using items normally found around the house or in a pharmacy. The following are some ideas to get you started:

lubricant
tongue depressor
rolls of gauze
old clothes that can be cut off from patients body
razor for erotic shaving

clothes-pins for pinching nipples, vulva, penis or scrotum

small flash light

flexible, overhead desk light to mimic an examination light

ice cubes and/or a warming device (e.g. fondue pot to change the temperature of medical instruments)

A more thorough doctor may also want to include items that are rather specialized, which may require the purchase of supplies from a sex toy shop or medical equipment supplier:

speculum

dildos, vibrators and butt plugs of varying sizes

strap on for dildo/vibrator

spreader bars to mimic stirrups at a doctor's office

Wartenberg pin-wheel (hand-held device, with wheel which has evenly spaced radiating sharp pins - rotates around as it is rolled across the flesh)

Enema kit

Crepe bandages are available in almost any first aid kit and they are surprisingly effective when used to restrain a patient, they are also comfortable to wear when applied flat against the skin, tight but not over-tight. Crepe bandage can be used to immobilise a joint, restrain a limb to a fixed object or limb to limb. Bandaging can be to one area of the body only or almost total coverage and total control and combined with other medical procedures and gadgets: catheters and tubes particularly come to mind... The crepe binding can be removed by unwinding or cut away using round ended scissors. Head bandages make for a great invisible man fantasy.

Sometimes you can find needles and cheap rubber gloves on sale. I also have glass-sucking-cups and and a liquid disinfectant also enables me to clean and then use other hot items. I also have some breathing-masks, the ones that cover the nose and mouth and then have a tube to breath through. These can be nicely combined with Saran wrap-mummies.

Costumes can be as simple as a lab coat or a loose fitting patient's gown. Sexy nurse outfits can easily be put together at home e.g. white zip up dress with matching bra and panties or a demure button up blouse and skirt with racy black lingerie underneath, white cap, white thigh-high stockings. I have a pair of 50's black heavy rimmed glasses that we used to call "birth control glasses" because they are so very unsexy. Alternatively, it is easy to use a ready-made nurse, dentist, or doctor's outfit purchased from adult or costume store. Remember that this is just icing the cake. A private room with a bed, a perhaps a white lab coat, and you are all ready for your check-up.

Many people shy away from role playing because they feel embarrassed, or worry that they will look or sound stupid. Contrary to this belief, a few keys phrases can act as wonderful ice breakers and magical momentum makers and are often all it takes to get into character and get the fun rolling, at which point who really cares? Get into the spirit of a medical fantasy with phrases like:

Do you want your naughty nurse to take a closer look?

Normally this procedure does not hurt, but since you have not been following doctor's orders...

Now I just want you to lay back and open your legs up wide so I can really take a look. If there is anything I can do to help you relax...

I am going to perform a treatment to help with your libido problem. I have been working on special technique called a medically induced Orgasm.

To maintain momentum as your play progresses, try saying:

Don't be embarrassed about the things I have to do to you. I want to reassure you I am a professional; this is not sexual for me at all, really!

Most of my male patients get hard-ons when it comes to this point in the exam. I do not mind. It is a compliment, especially coming from you.

Doctor, it still hurts real bad. I need you to lift up my skirt again and take another look.

When you think about things you say during a role play, consider it more like witty banter, rather than cheesy dialogue. The point is to establish some common ground for your shared fantasy, to try and keep a straight face while you say or do something that ups the tension and keeps your partner guessing! A great way to come up with more dialogue ideas is to read up on erotica that centres around your role play fantasy of choice. The more you become familiar with the type of language used, the easier and more natural it will feel to embody your role.

To begin with you might want to try the on-duty fantasy. You are a doctor and nurse in a busy hospital. One of you is in a white jacket, the other in nurse's uniform. It has been a hard night and as the nurse passes the doctor's room, the doctor calls out:

"You look worn out. Got a headache?"

"Yes, doctor. I can't seem to get rid of it."

"Well, I know a cure for that, nurse. Hop up on the couch and I'll give you a neck massage." Nurse lies down and the doctor says: "I'm really good at relieving tension this way, nurse. Just tell me if this feels good."

"Oh doctor, you do have healing hands."

As the doctor strokes the nurse's neck, one hand strays down to other parts of the body.

"You're really tense, nurse, you should have a proper massage, you know. I read in an old medical book that this can help."

The doctor then produces a feather and/or vibrator, and gently unbuttons the nurse's uniform. The doctor then gently strokes the nurse's nipples, belly and genitals, with either feather or vibrator or both.

"Does this feel better?"

"Oh yes, doctor. But it really does feel tense here...and here...and here."

Since the metal of a stethoscope is cold and hard you can have great fun putting it on sensitive body parts like nipples and buttocks. But if your local fancy dress shop does not have one, try this: get the nurse to close her eyes and use the back of a cold spoon instead.

There is a whole sexual subculture enjoyed by people who like to give each other 'thorough medical examinations'. Hire some surgical greens from a fancy dress shop, invest in surgical gloves and experiment with ever more invasive procedures.

Go through a flirty triage routine. Ask him some basic questions about his health and about the reason for his visit. Are there any areas that he is specifically concerned about? Allow your breasts to 'accidentally' settle around his arm or brush his shoulder while you check his pulse. Help him get his shoes off, affording a glance down your shirt, but be sure that you catch him looking and that you make eye contact briefly and give him a subtle, knowing little smile: something that says "I know you were checking me out, but I'll let it go because I think you're cute." Ask him to remove his clothing, and give him a Snuggie or a towel or something akin to a hospital gown to change into. Leave the room while he changes.

There will be a noticeable bulge in his "gown" when you re-enter the room. Notice it, but be cute about noticing it. It is the elephant in the room that neither of you can acknowledge. Yet.

Ask him to lay back and extend his arms. Pick an arm and manipulate the area from his shoulder to his fingertips, slowly. Ostensibly, you are checking range of motion, sensitivity, looking for lifestyle and pathological manifestations like track marks, inflamed lymph nodes, cysts, etc... Make it obvious that you enjoy touching his arms, and say something that suggests that you noticed that he works out.

Position his arm so that it is in contact with your body in the most suggestive way possible, without being completely obvious. Tuck his hand and wrist between your arm and side while you are checking him out so that he feels like he is getting away with a bit of a "feel."

He will be dying for oral sex by now. He has called your "bluff" in his head, and will expect you to ditch the act and get to it. Do not do it yet. Tell him to lay his arms at his sides. Observe the general shape of the abdomen, noting any distension, irregularity, or abnormality. Look for discolouration of the skin, and be sure to ask about any scars you notice. Ask about them in a sexy way, though: "I'll bet there's a REALLY interesting story behind THIS scar" for example. He will have one.

Palpate and percuss his abdomen as though you had any clue as to how to identify something like an inflamed liver or discern between the sound of a healthy or terminally ill GI tract. Tell him you need to consult with the doctor, or check with the doctor, or whatever. Leave the room for a couple minutes.

Return and apologize for the doctor's absence, but tell your "patient" that there are still some tests you can (and need) to do.

Advise him that you are going to check for hernia. He will really bite down when you say that, because he will be thinking you are going to go to town now.

Open the bottom of his gown, exposing his genitals. Hide your grin. It is important that you maintain the iciest of affects while you examine him. Start with one ball (choose your favourite) and give it a thorough working-over. Do the same for the other ball, or balls (depending on your man's build). Be sure to get your face close enough that he can feel the warmth of your breath, but do not do anything sexual. Give them a once-over for testicular cancer, too.

Now put on a very concerned look. Think of the last time you were in a hospital waiting-room expecting the worst news about your dad. Tell your boyfriend you need to talk to the doctor and then vanish as quickly as possible.

Make him wait at least 10 minutes.

Return with a large, glass thermometer and a tub of Vaseline. Tell your boyfriend to turn onto his stomach. Tell him that you forgot to take his temperature and that it is imperative that you get his core temp ASAP. Slather the thermometer with lube and cram it up your man's butt.

Yes, I just said that.

Wait at least 5 minutes, without saying anything. If he tries to engage you in conversation, be dismissive. Pull the thermometer out, look at it (holding it obviously away from your face), frown, and then leave the room for approximately 5 minutes.

Return with the same lube and a rubber glove. Tell him to assume the "duck and cover" position: ass up, knees on the table, elbows on the table, fingers intertwined over the back of the head. Advise him that he might feel some initial discomfort, but that you are a nurse and you know exactly what you are doing. Apply a liberal amount of lube to your index and middle fingers. Going slowly, enter your boyfriend and locate his prostate. Massage it until full release has occurred.

For something less invasive, imagine that you are sick and confined to bed. These days, very few doctors make house calls, but remember, this is a fantasy! In this scenario, your personal physician is happy to show up bedside to check up on you. But it turns out he or she has some unorthodox ideas on patient care. In specific, the doctor believes strongly in the power of sexual healing. You still cannot leave the bed. Doctor's orders! Just lie back and let the doctor take care of things, starting with a very thorough examination. Remember, this is all for your own good.

Alternatively, it is time for your annual examination and as luck would have it, you have a very thorough and attentive primary care doctor at your disposal. He or she wants to make sure every part of your body is fit and healthy. If you find yourself getting aroused during the exam, well, that is natural. Your doctor is a professional, surely he or she has seen it before. Fortunately for you, it turns out your doctor believes in being very hands-on when it comes to relieving patient discomfort. Is your examining nurse naive and unaware of how her charms are spilling over the collar of her blouse, or is she a naughty nurse intent on seduction? Was that flash of panty glimpsed under a short white skirt intentional? You decide if a hand brushing the patient's crotch is an innocent mistake or a calculated move. Now who is seducing who? This is very standard porno plot. Some more adventurous types might want to try something a little more adventurous.

In a medical situation we are conditioned to be submissive; we position our bodies as we are told and our replies to the questions we are asked determine the treatment that we are to receive. The treatment prescribed may be humiliating or painful but we are conditioned to accept it because it will make us better. This domination/submission situation and its sexual overtones are exploited when playing the role of patient to a fantasy doctor or nurse. The examination is designed to humiliate the submissive patient: this is emphasised by requiring the patient to strip off all clothing and jewellery All army recruits - and martial artists - are familiar with a medical examination intended to check their fitness to fight. It is a cross between an army medical and a strip search. They start off stripped to the waist for a chest examination and finish up fully-naked. A doctor with a sadistic attitude can make it a memorably humiliating procedure. There is complete body examination including detailed cock and balls examination and a rectal examination. They may also have to answer questions about their sex life - when most recently penetrated orally and anally and the frequency and times of masturbation. During the course of the examination the naked patient is required to move into humiliating positions, the examination includes touching the patient externally, including intimate areas such as the arm pits and genitals, and then internally at all orifices. An involuntary erection may result in further humiliation of the naked male patient. The medical profession has many instruments with which to invade the body of a patient and equipment designed to hold the patient securely yet humiliatingly open to examination. Simple procedures can be administered in a humiliating manner to the fully-naked patient: vital signs - core temperature (measured rectally) and blood pressures; mouth washing under close supervision, administration of rectal suppositories and enemas. Reactions can be tested, body hair shaved and samples required of all body fluids. Reflexes can be tested: in particular the subject can be trained to control his gag reflex by being able to accept two or more latex-gloved fingers in his mouth and deep in his throat. This will also test the production of saliva. Pain thresholds, pain masking and resistance to pain may be tested.

For sportsmen, the aerobic threshold may be measured and endurance testing recommended if time and suitable equipment is available. A good starting point is for the patient to be required to drink a litre (two pints) of plain water at the beginning of the examination, but to be forbidden to pass it until specifically told to pass it as a sample, under observation. This can include checking that the patient can stop and restart the flow on command. Some common medical symptoms might include: groin pain, night emissions - wet dreams, poor eyesight, tight scrotum and itching foreskin.

16. Drugs and Aphrodisiacs

In a world of sexual fantasy, there is no need for real life pharmaceuticals of any kind. The human brain is powerful enough to create its own higher states of conciousness. The placebo effect is well known to scientists all over the world and works equally well in the bedroom. Any common candy can take the place of the most potent pills and a partner can be informed that a simple glass of red wine has been laced with the strongest aphrodisiac known to man. Psychedelic drugs such as GHB, ecstasy and ketamine have all kinds of legal ramifications. It is much more fun if you can get her all worked up on a placebo. These days supplements come in really funky capsules. I recently saw a bag of sample tasters, which included a golden creatine capsule, a red metallic caffeine capsule and a blue/silver 'sexual performance' capsule. The last one was mostly mostly maca with a few other herbs so there is little chance of even spacing out let alone overdosing.

If the female partner wishes to be more involved in the role play. Then the idea of a a sexually cold woman, captured, who hates you and is forced to drink an aphrodisiac can be a good starting point. You then wait. Soon, she begins to feel its effects. She insults you. She hates you, but, too, it is apparent that she will soon need you, desperately, sexually. She attempts to fight the effects of the aphrodisiac, both verbally and by body movements, trying to resist it. She is, of course, unable to do so. Then she agrees, haughtily, condescendingly, to go to bed with you. You refuse. She is shocked. She had not counted on this. The drug continues to work in her system, relentlessly. Soon she begs you to make love to her. Still, you refuse. Then, desperately, she realizes she must provoke you sexually. She strips herself. She moves before you. She, at last, helpless in the piteous crisis of her need, kneels before you, her hair over your feet, pleading that you make love to her. You give her permission to make love to you. She begins by kissing your feet, moving with her lips and touch lasciviously all the way up your body. At this point you carry her to the bed, and there let her continue to attempt to please you sexually. When you are satisfied that has suffered enough you turn her about and, to her joy, engage with her in mutual caressings, until together your needs are both satisfied. This requires an excellent female actress. The burden of the performance is on her. Psychologically, incidentally, this is an excellent fantasy for the female in two respects. First, in feeling herself into the role, and imagining what it would be like to be overwhelmed by powerful sexual feelings, which are not answered by those of another, detailed awareness of the nature of her sexual arousal, in terms of sensation and desire, are required.

The 'fake' aspects of being aroused is an interesting learning experience in self awareness. It is paying attention to what it like is to completely want a man. This is healthy for a woman who wants to enlarge and intensify her sexual appetites, bringing them more into the open, increasing their clarity. If she speaks what is theoretically occurring in her body, this can be of equal importance to the male partner who wishes to learn more about the feelings and emotions of his lover. Many men have very little notion of the sexual sensations, the inner life, of the female's body, either in arousal or orgasm. For example, does she feel a warmth in arousal? Are there sensations in her breasts, and along the sides of her body? What does a clitoral erection feel like? Are there incipient pelvic movements? Are there incipient vaginal contractions? What does it feel like to the woman when her vagina loosens and becomes sweet with the oils that make penetration such a delight, inviting it so eagerly? This just goes to show that pretend arousal can induce, through psychological techniques, arousal. It is hard to pretend you are sexually excited, particularly in a sexually exciting situation, without actually becoming sexually excited. A second psychological benefit for the woman is that it puts her, for at least once in her life, in a position that is only too painfully familiar to the male; that is, the position of the one who, though cruelly aroused, can be refused, repudiated and left unsatisfied. It would be well for her to have this painful and humiliating experience at least once in her life, even though it is in play. It is quite possible that it will make a better lover as well as a more understanding, human being out of her.

For the male, of course, this can be a delightful fantasy. Here he, in a delicious turnabout, finds that it is he, and not she, who is in the position to either answer or not answer desperately aroused sexual needs. She, of course, cannot overpower him. She can only beg him to satisfy her needs. Here the male can sense the sexual power of a woman, in choosing to bestow or not bestow, her sexual favours. He can see her delight in teasing him, putting him aside, evading him, playing with him, making him squirm before her in his need. These are not always pleasant gratifications, but they can be delicious to a woman. Now, in this fantasy, it is she who is put in the place of the male as their victim; it is he who can make her squirm, as women have made men squirm in the millions for thousands of years, perhaps since the abolition of capture as a mating institution. What man exists who would not, in the bottom of his heart, if only in a vengeance of his sex, relish the sight of a woman kneeling at his feet, begging him to make love to her.

Commercially advertised aphrodisiacs are probably best avoided. They are at best either useless or dangerous. The stimulations here must be mental, not chemical. Contrary to popular opinion Viagra is not an aphrodisiac. It is physical stimulant with unpleasant side effects and little fine control. This is not a book for men with physical performance issues. If you wish to use an actual substance, a glass of wine is an excellent idea. Women like wine; it is 'sexy' to them; it relaxes them; it makes them glow; it lowers their inhibitions. Only a small amount of wine, however, perhaps a glass or two is necessary. Being drunk does not improve sexual performance. Alcohol, chemically, is actually an anaesthetic.

Sex, particularly imaginative sex, calls for the brain to be fully active. It wants the physical and intellectual powers performing at their very peak. Similarly, it is not a good idea to have sex when you are drowsy, weary or sleepy. Sex, is terrific, and is well worth being wide awake for. Setting aside an hour or two in the morning or the afternoon is not a bad idea; then, the children may be in school, and the entire home will be at your disposal, increasing the range of your sexual activities considerably. If the daylight hours are not practical, then the early evening is a good time. If your children are very young, you can make love shortly after they are asleep; if they are older, just tell them you wish to make love and lock the bedroom door; you can always see them for a snack before they go to bed. There is nothing wrong with children knowing that their parents love one another; they must be taught to respect their parents, just as all the books teach us to respect them. Children will probably have a much healthier attitude toward sex if they know that Mommy is happily being had by Daddy in the next room, than if they hide sex. We can tell tell children as much as we like that sex is healthy but if we do not act in an appropriate fashion, why should they ever believe us? What we do means much more than what we say. Today, many kids think they know more about sex than their parents; it is not necessary that we conspire to perpetuate their delusion. 83% of U.S. teenagers have sex for the first time before receiving any formal sex education. When the youngsters realize that Mom and Dad are making out in the next room, they may be initially scandalized, but I expect, they will also be really proud of them. Why should Mom and Dad care what they think, any more than they care what Mom and Dad think? They will rightly be envious. They do not have anything so good going for them. In addition, the security and comfort of the bedroom in your own home beats the back seat of a Volvo, almost every time.

A last bit of embroidery on the aphrodisiac fantasy might be mentioned. After the woman has unequivocally yielded, passionately, putatively under the influence of the drug, you then inform her that she had been given only a placebo, that it had not been an aphrodisiac at all. Now she faces a dilemma. She has been tricked into revealing her true nature. She has been outwitted, tricked and forced to reveal herself as what she truly is, an incredibly passionate female. She can no longer lie. She lies nude and exposed to him, physically and psychologically. She has been truly had, both mentally and physically. The idea that her inner slut comes out merely by the power of suggestion is extremely enticing and will lead to some frank and interesting discussions later on when you show her that it was really was her all along. This in itself can bring a relationship to whole new levels.

17. Exotic Dancers and Sexy Strippers

To see a woman remove her clothing is an exciting experience. To watch her body moving provocatively, to rhythmic erotic music, is a treat and a delight. These days, a huge industry has grown out of this simple activity. The problem with the professional strip tease, of course, is that it is a rather glumly commercial, if not cynical, exhibition. It is mostly, not a fulfilling and satisfying, but a frustrating experience. Imagine instead the pleasure of being treated, privately, to this performance by an excited, loving woman, who is eager that you make love to her. As her performance concludes, she dances, lovingly and aroused, to your arms.

Dancing can be extremely subtle or wildly raucous depending on personal tastes. My own feeling is that the more jarring bumps and grinds seen on poles and stages may be less appropriate in the bedroom than on the athletic field. Some women can dance beautifully while scarcely moving. They have the music burning deep inside their bodies. Not all the clothing commonly worn by women can be removed gracefully. A wrap-around skirt is more easily removed, for example, than a pair of skin tight jeans. Hooks are more easily disengaged than buttons. Details and planning in this matter are best left to the lady. Allow her to surprise you with her erotic inventiveness.

Despite the fact that pole dancing is now an Olympic sport, most women have very little experience when it comes to strip tease. One useful tip that works well in the privacy of your own home is for the dancer to approach the spectator and assist in the very last part of any removal. She might teasingly slide off a glove and allow him to pull away the very last ten percent. Seductively draping items over him works well, as does flinging items at him for added effect.

Perhaps it is the fact that I am a man that I feel that male strippers are over-rated. I have never really been a fan of female strippers perhaps with the exception of Grace Jones as Katrina in the the wonderful movie Vamp, who took erotic dancing to a new level of artistic performance. Perhaps I simply have not been exposed to enough strippers to become a connoisseur. The only time that I have seen male strippers has been in The Full Monty and on the UK Channel 4 documentary entitled appropriately enough Confessions of a Male Stripper: First Cut. Neither depictions were particularly glamorous but I am pleased to tell you that away from the money obsessed club scene, a man putting on a few moves for a woman who is already interested can be a very exciting experience. Many of the same guidelines apply to males as they do to females. My advice is to choose items like hats and robes, as removing socks and trousers is not very erotic and requires an incredible sense of balance.

For females, a belly dancer's costume is extremely enticing, especially if she wears a veil, which is only torn aside when she is thrown to her back on the bed. Armlets, bangles and bells all add to the effect. The sound of these bells, as she responds to you, can be highly stimulating. Some writers have claimed that belly dancing is one of humankind's greatest inventions, somewhere between fire and the wheel. It is impossible for a female to learn to belly dance and still not know what being a female is all about. It trains her body in the motions of love and makes her graceful, sensuous and beautiful. It makes her exotic, delicious, provocative, desirable. It drives men crazy with lust. Many women have an interest in being desirable, beautiful and dangerously, deliciously erotic. They wish, sometimes, to be as stimulating and sexy as they can. And it is hard to be sexier than when belly dancing. It is an invention made to combine movement, music, beauty and sex. Barefoot, in bangles, vulnerable in the revealing costume of the belly dancer, almost any woman becomes an incredibly exciting sexual object. There are also, of course, all sorts of enriching sexual overtones involved in such a performance. It is almost as if she were a woman of another culture, conditioned to please the senses of men. Perhaps she is a woman of another culture, a culture in which women are permitted to be little more than the servants or slaves of males? Perhaps she is a western woman, a captive or slave in a harem or brothel, trained and forced to perform these dances, say, for customers, or for her master? Is she alone, or are there others, too? How does she compare with them? Is she beaten if she does not perform satisfactorily? Are gold coins thrown to her feet, which she must pick up and carry quickly to her master?

If you happen to own an oriental rug, that, presumably, would be the most desirable place for her to dance. The evidence seems to suggest that frequent and joyful sex is good for you. It is not unhealthy to use the human body for its most important purpose. In this case, why not give up one of more destructive habits such as smoking or drinking and instead use the money to send your partner to a belly dancing class. If this is not possible, due to location then check on the internet for video instructions.

As an interesting alternative to this fantasy is that of the dancer at an 'anything goes' nightclub. As a special promotion, the club has sponsored a drawing; the winner gets full and complete use of the stripper for an evening, and the stripper must allow the winner to do whatever he or she wants. The winner takes full advantage of the prize, using the stripper as a sex toy; the stripper must be completely obedient and allow the winner to do whatever the winner wishes, regardless of how the stripper feels about it.

A twist on this scenario is the fan letter. This fantasy is like playing the lottery and your chances of winning are real. Many men dream to being with an adult model for a day. The good news is that some performers have a personal page and a forum where they interact with the fans. Once a month they pick one lucky guy. You can build up to this by beginning with some email correspondence. Send your partner some fan mail, telling her what you like most about her. Go to town on the descriptions, tell her your favourite roles that you have seen her play in various porn films. Talk about what you have seen her do and in turn what you would like to do to her. Whether you write like a gentleman or a sex crazed pig and a stalker is completely up to you.

Have her reply to your email, informing you that you have won a special evening with the actress herself. This will be your opportunity to make all those fantasies come true.

18. FAMILY AFFAIRS

Incest fantasies are surprisingly common even though most people who experience them are horrified by thoughts of actual sex with their relatives. Many women would like to try the father/daughter role play but have never had any inappropriate thoughts about their actual fathers Most would think of the reality as gross. This means that it is a subject that even the closest of lovers are usually embarrassed to raise.

If as a couple, you can overcome this societal stigma, these fantasies can be extremely rewarding, partly because they are so forbidden. In many of our modern nanny states, the boogey-man of child abuse is something that the media revels in blowing completely out of proportion. In most countries, the Child Protection Services is far less accountable than the police or other branches of the public services and have far reaching powers that put the fear of god into ordinary parents. This is despite the fact that child kidnapping is an extremely rare occurrence. Statistically speaking a child is one hundred times more likely to be involved in a fatal car accident than being snatched from the street. Of course this does not prevent over zealous bureaucrats from prosecuting parents who allow their children to walk home from school unaccompanied, as recently happened in Maryland.

If you think that incest is taboo in porn, then you are clearly not watching enough porn! Despite such a clear taboo there is still all sorts of mother/daughter, father/son and twin/sibling stuff out there. Although most of it tends to revolve around step-parents and step-siblings, (at least that is what I have heard...) it is still popular. Perhaps it is porn that pushes the boundaries and opens people's eyes to different fantasies.

The recent rash of scandals involving celebrities and allegations of abuse has given the subject an undue amount of sensational media attention. A number of individuals have been viciously scape-goated, although none of the root causes have been addressed. Let us keep this in its proper context. What goes on the privacy of a couple's bedroom is sacrosanct. It is a pale of imagination and experimentation and as long as both parties are consenting, anything should be acceptable.

In many cases it is the taboo that is the attraction. The lust to break the rules and to defy the taboo is the attraction. Ask any woman who has lusted after her room mate's boyfriend Ask any any man who was inappropriately aroused by a prepubescent Christina Ricci in The Addams Family or Christina Applegate in Married With Children - taboo relationships are hot. These feelings are strongest when there is a lot of reluctance and agonizing over the wrongness of the act but the need to have just one hot forbidden episode is just too much for them to stop themselves. Some people actually enjoy the fact that there is an element of repulsion that needs to be overcome. It makes everything more raw.

In Brett Kahr's book, Who's Been Sleeping in Your Head? The Secret World of Sexual Fantasies, Kahr, a British psychotherapist, explores this same controversy. His work, based on extensive research with a non-clinical population, shows the surprising range of disturbing, frightening and challenging fantasies that exist in the heads of people that are living healthy, successful lives. One of the most surprising was the tale of an older Jewish woman, whose parents had died in the Holocaust. And yet this grandmotherly woman revealed that her most powerful orgasms came to fantasies of her being sexually examined and abused by Nazis, while strapped nude to a surgical table.

I recently had a girlfriend that was nearly twenty years younger than me. She would would call me when she was drunk and insist I pick her up and take her 'home' from the bar. I always knew she was drunk and not just calling to say hello because she called me Papa when I answered. She wanted me to act angry and scold her and play this stern father figure. This got her really worked up. she would often go out in a Catholic schoolgirl type outfit which was fun. It was odd at first, but I easily got into the act.

In the typical daddy/daughter fantasy, either party can play the role of seducer. For some it is an exciting extension of teacher student role plays. The daughter might come home from class with a bad report card and daddy teaches her a rough lesson. Of course this is wrong in real life but this is a world of fantasy and that is part of what makes it so exciting for some people. Squeals of 'No Daddy, please!' can ignite some of our most primal passions in both parties. Of course the

"Daddy, you shouldn't be doing this!" protestations can always be reversed with the female taking the role of Lolita.

"Sweety, what on earth are you doing naked in my bed? Go to your room right now before your mummy finds out."

"Don't worry Daddy, she is gone for the weekend."

In one well documented case, a wife asked her husband to pretend to be her father during sex, and to pretend to molest her. The husband was worried this might be based on a true event in his wife's past, and what was he supposed to do? How could he help his wife? Was this normal or healthy? It was suggested that this fantasy might be a way in which the wife the wife was re-establishing control over her sexuality, and recovering from a history of trauma. This is an interesting point and flips the issue on its head. The fantasy is not a symptom of an illness, but is instead an adaptive effort to overcome a history of trauma and re-assume control of one's mind and life.

The Electra complex is the other side of the coin for girls - who love daddy too much and/or got mixed messages from daddy (and, sometimes, mom) about dad's availability. It gets played out all the time, in the 'dance' of the younger woman who is 'hot' for the older guy. Real world father/daughter relationships can have a definite impact on the popularity of such fantasies. It has been reported for example that in Asian Confucian cultures, a parental bias towards sons leaves daughters feeling left out and even unloved. Therefore in some situations the father daughter fantasy is extremely strong. Many Chinese girls are incredibly attracted to the daddy/daughter scenario and love nothing better than being bent over a lover's knee until their behinds are spanked red raw while being given stern lectures. When they are told that they would be punished even more harshly if their mother ever found out what a little slut she was, it just adds to the excitement. Not everybody's cup of tea but for some, extremely arousing.

I once met a sexy Singaporean girl as a cosplay convention that really wanted me to dress up as Darth Vader. I think that she had serious daddy issues, and so I made her buy a slave Leia costume. The combination of costumes and incest was incredible and resulted in some of the wildest sex that I have ever experienced.

The mother/son dynamic is generally much less explored by most couples, even though the Oedipal complex is a popular subject in academic circles. Jamie Lee Curtis in the movie 'Bad Mother' is often referenced as the epitome of this wickedness of the mother breaking the taboo for the boy. Another much more common form of 'seduction' by the mother is to 'keep her all to herself', thus, we have the momma's boy. As it is easy to become accustomed to being taken care of, the son can become irredeemably lazy; with plenty of woman hatred perking and the accompanying psychological trauma.

Sometimes this is just an 'Older woman, take me in hand!' fantasy. There is good reason why The Graduate still holds up – up to a certain age, that is. It seems every "boy" wants his Mrs. Robinson to show him the ropes. And the ladies? Are they imagining their responsibilities guiding and mentoring, for the future benefit of other women? Some women really enjoy the young boy, older woman fantasy. Something about how teenage boys are just walking erections and the thought of seeing a naked breast makes them go crazy, and how a woman lowers herself so much to let one of those kids have her. She is risking so much just to get some young hard dick. And his dick probably isn't even that big yet.

The last variation that I want to discuss here is the brother/sister fantasy. It has been on the decline as the size of families have decreased over time. In an age when there are so many single child families, many youngsters have never had the opportunity to fantasise sexually about an older sibling. For others, this is a very common fantasy. Imagine a situation when a young boy is caught by his sister enjoying some illicit porn. At first she acts all high and mighty even though she is of a

104

similar age to start being intrigued by sexual subjects. As she becomes more and more excited she at the same time time keeps insisting that this is wrong. It does not take long before she takes on the role of seductress. How many teenage boys have fantasised being interrupted by an older sister, and rather than them being appalled, having them offering to lend a helping hand.

Game of Thrones author George R. R. Martin regularly includes a good helping of incest into his fantasy novels. In a recent interview he explained, "Well, you can't marry your sister anymore, but I'm sure there are people who still sleep with them." He simply laughs off the fact that some people object to this kind of thing "There are a million books out there, which is my reaction when I get one of these letters. You don't happen to like a lot of sex in your fantasy, then there are 37 other authors you could read who don't have sex in their fantasy. Have fun. It's an important part of human life and necessary for any kind of realistic portrayal. That's my audience. It's a sad commentary on American morals that the sex is the thing that people object to. I find that sad, but it is true. I can describe an axe entering a person's skull and no one objects, but if I describe a penis entering a vagina, there's an outcry."

19. KIDNAPPED

The Kidnap Fantasy is a common one for many women and it can be performed and elaborated in a number of exciting ways. I have one lady friend that likes nothing more that being taken prisoner by vicious, brutal warlords. She enjoys being tied up and subjected to a wide variety of sexual tortures immensely, with her own unique kink being that a fellow hostage is executed every time she reaches orgasm. Unsurprisingly, her orgasm always came extremely quickly and in very rapid succession.

In the real world, Stockholm syndrome is a phenomenon in which hostages develop positive feelings toward their captors. This is perhaps because they are forced to undergo such enormous psychological and emotional stresses. When I was younger many of my fellow scuba instructors were drawn to the profession not because of the tropical locations or underwater beauty but because there were so many opportunities to rescue panicking beauties as they underwent a potentially life threatening situation. The bond that this created with their instructors led to many brief but intense holiday romances. Not many forms of employment have such interesting perks.

This on the other hand is simply a kidnapping fantasy and yet a realistic role play can have interesting and long lasting effects. This is analogous to the individual who, in real life, is quite shy and reticent, but, given a role, as in a play, can throw himself into it with élan and gusto, and perform with a realism that startles everyone. Many genuinely gifted actors are rather introverted, quiet individuals. Often they cannot easily be recognized from role to role, they are so gifted. This is very different from the average Hollywood star. The success of people like Nicholas Cage and Russell Crowe usually depend upon them playing themselves over and again over under different names. One of the general attractions and strengths of imaginative sex is that it provides individuals with roles. People who do not know what to do in their own person, or are afraid to do anything in their own person, can often perform superbly in the context of playing a role. Indeed, some people live life as a set of roles. These sexual fantasies can be extremely cathartic and can occasionally reproduce the reactions that are common in very high stress situations.

A good introduction to the kidnapping fantasy is for one partner to inconspicuously follow the other. My own partner becomes very excited knowing that I am watching her from a distance, keeping a very close eye on her, sizing her up as a desirable victim for a sexual kidnapping. This works well while she is shopping down town and I trail her movements. There is something very exciting about observing her and stalking her, which perhaps harks back to our days as hunter-gatherers. She too finds it be a delicious thrill, moving about innocently, as though she were completely unaware, yet knowing that I am somewhere near, following her, observing her. If you both have a car, you might even try following her on the public roads. Maybe she notices, in the rear-view mirror, that another car seems to be following hers? She is slightly puzzled but decides to think nothing of it and dismisses it from her mind.

The actual capture need not be done outside. Indeed this would probably be inviting the wrong kind of attention completely. Instead that action can take place at night, in her bedroom. She can remain fully clothed or roughly stripped at gun point, the choice is yours. If you are role playing with a weapon, it is best to leave it home even if it is fake. Some people feel a temptation to do it like Bonnie and Clyde, but guns and knives are as phallic as they are dangerous. Real weapons do not belong in play - you could wind up having the bad kind of mind-blowing sex. Get a toy version if you are planning to mess around.

She is bound and gagged, and taken to the car. She kneels on the floor, crouched over in the foot well of the front seat. A blanket is thrown over her to conceal her body. Then, around town and through traffic, stopping for lights, she is driven to her captors hideaway. After thirty minutes or so he takes her to 'his place.' 'His place,' of course, is once again the bedroom. In this fantasy she may wish to be blindfolded, or have a sack tied over her head. It is removed, if at all, only when she finds herself in the 'strange bed.' If she wishes, everything could take place while she is blindfolded, or has a sack fastened over her head and tied about her neck. After all, providing she has not seen him before that time, she will not be able to recognize him later. After the fantasy is completed, the partners may then pretend that he has placed her, hooded, nude, bound hand and foot, in some public place, where she will be found in the morning. In such a case she would never even have seen her assailant.

In this fantasy, the captive must not be placed in the trunk of the car. That does not provide her with sufficient air. Furthermore, if a sack is tied over the head it must be of some material through which air easily filters. Under no circumstances should an airtight bag, for example, a plastic bag, be used.

An alternative hostage scenario is to use a little prior planning and arrange a night in a seedy motel at the edge of town. The victim is driving innocently through town and stops at a set of traffic lights, when a desperate criminal opens the passenger door and gets into the car. He proceeds to car-jack the victim's car in order to escape from pursuing police forces. The driver is forced at gun or knifepoint to drive to a seedy motel on the edge of town, where he or she decides to take advantage of the turn of events by raping the victim in the run-down motel room.

Kidnapping offers a great many opportunities for complex elaboration. Perhaps she is a wealthy heiress, snatched by the local mafia in order to extract a hefty ransom from her rich industrialist father. I actually had the opportunity to play out this game with a girl whose father was in real life a leading factory owner in the area. She revelled in the pre-planning and the details of the set up. We cut out letters from a magazine to create an anonymous ransom note and once she had finished glueing them onto the paper, she practically exploded with passion. I have never before or since seen such a prim and proper young lady turn into such an animalistic, wanton hussy. I had unwittingly unleashed a storm of pent up sexuality which I shall never forget.

20. MASTERS AND SLAVES

The subjugated sex slave is one of the most provocative sexual fantasies that a man and a woman can share. It answers a deep male desire to own and dominate a woman but at the same time it also answers to a woman's instinctive desire to be owned and dominated. It is important here to understand that we are acting out fantasies here not stating immutable biological laws. Although such carnal desires clearly exist, they do so alongside many others. For example, the male also desires to respect and love the woman; and the woman also desires, paradoxically, to be independent and free. The strength of these relative desires doubtless varies considerably from individual to individual. Each human being is unique. Many of us share the same sexual fantasies but we are different in many other ways. This can certainly be seen in external anatomical appearances with so many different body shapes, sizes, colours and types. You might also be surprised to learn that we also have considerable internal differences which remain invisible to the outside world. Organ sizes are by no means standard and even a key feature such as the heart can have a varying number of valves coming into it. With so much physical difference, it makes sense that there will also be considerable psychological divergence. In terms of emotional capacities and neurological dispositions we are all very much individuals. Not to mention environmental forces and cultural influences. We now understand that gender is not black and white, but a vast spectrum of possibilities. This can be seen in the more liberal nations where heterosexuals, homosexuals, bisexuals and even transsexuals are openly tolerated. My own personal preference is that of a trisexual: I will try anything once.

Despite this huge palette of colours from which to chose, the master and slave is a regularly recurring theme. For many of us, nothing so excites a man as to have a woman admit herself his slave, his to do with as he wishes. Similarly, nothing so excites a woman as to feel herself his slave, to feel herself his, and to know that she must do what he tells her. Despite its apparent simplicity it represents sexuality of great subtlety and complexity.

The key to any sexual encounter is consent. Sado-masochism is only violence by metaphor: a closer metaphor would be to view sadomasochism as theatre. Practitioners use terms such as 'top and bottom' or 'dominant and submissive', but never 'victim and assailant', which emphasises the fact that both partners are active in the encounter, albeit in different roles. Just as in straight sex, the only difference between a loving act and a violent act is consent. Any sexual acts is an act of violence if it is undertaken without consent. Consenting sexual acts have absolutely nothing to do with violence. This is not about exploitation and degradation. The man who truly abuses a woman is not a man. He is no more than the monster who abuses animals or children. Indeed many people 'switch', that is take different roles at different times. Sado-masochism (the technical term for master and slave fantasies) is essentially a ritual, there are ritualised stop words, even the most tyrannical practitioner knows where not to hit hard and usually knows a great deal more about human anatomy than the average man in the street. The bottoms outnumber the tops at least ten to one, and the bottoms in reality dominate the ritual. One of the most important rules ... is that the bottom sets the limits to the encounter. The result is an intense form of erotic gratification which by its very nature involves levels of trust and compassion rarely found in any other walks of life.

When practised properly, sexual fantasy of any kind requires that you respect your partner's wants, desires, expectations, and limitations. Those who engage in safe and consensual master and slave relationships have much to teach the rest of us about what consent really means. Within the this context, consent is not merely the absence of 'no,' but a far more qualitative conversation that involves negotiation, the sharing of fantasies and the setting of limits.

It must be noted though that in legal terms the situation is often far less clear. A number of recent cases show that prejudices, fear and ignorance can lead to injustice. In a case dubbed 'Paddleboro' by journalists, police in Attleboro, Massachusetts raided a BDSM (bondage, discipline, and sadomasochism) private party and arrested both the host and a guest who paddled another woman with a large wooden kitchen spoon, allegedly causing bruising and bleeding. The case immediately sparked controversy over the limits of sexual freedom and caused fear among those in the S/M community that they would be targeted by law enforcement. Lawyers for the defendants argued that the state should not be prosecuting the accused for assault and battery, especially when the victim did not complain. Despite this fact, the state insisted on going forward with the prosecution anyway. From the press reports, the prosecution seems motivated by politics, not protection. This demonstrates the legal restraints on violence may, in fact, undermine individual liberty. This sort of overreaching and sexual repression is not an isolated instance. In a UK case, widely known as Operation Spanner, the court ruled that consent was not a valid legal defence for wounding and actual bodily harm. Even though every one present at the S/M party was a willing participant in the activities, the police and Crown Prosecution Service insisted on pressing charges and sixteen men were charged with various offences, including assault occasioning actual bodily harm. In a prime example of institutionalised homophobia, even the submissives were convicted of 'aiding and abetting,' for the crime of consenting to their own injuries. Because the activities included erotic piercing, some body art professionals are still worried that UK judges can interpret their practices as illegal, determining which consensual acts are too extreme and constitute assault, on a case-by-case basis, with no way of the practitioner knowing beforehand. The most well known artist present, Alan Oversby, also known as Mr Sebastian, was charged with assault, occasioning actual bodily harm for performing a genital piercing on a client. He was also charged with using anaesthetic without a licence and for sending obscene material through the post (photographs of piercings).

This kind of prosecution only succeeds in driving such activities underground. Forced to carry on furtively and illegally, sado-masochists who will be unable to meet openly and obtain recommendations about responsible partners will be at much greater risk from real violence. The community will not be able to inform newcomers about 'Tops' who are not safe and this will become a secret dangerous society. Neither the gay community or S/M practitioners will now come forward to the police because of fear of incriminating themselves.

In addition, this blatant discrimination against the gay community was especially clear in the infamous serial killer case of Jerry Dahmer. On May 27, 1991, two teenage cousins saw a young boy, whom they described as 'butt naked,' bleeding, and having difficulty speaking. The young women immediately called 911, and attempted to explain the situation to the police when they arrived. However, by this time Dahmer had arrived on the scene and the officers simply took him at his word that the fourteen-year-old Konerak was his nineteen-year-old lover. Speaking only to Dahmer and ignoring the attempts by Konerak to speak in Laotian, the police believed Dahmer when he said that Konerak had too much to drink and wandered naked into the street while Dahmer was out getting more beer. The cousins tried to explain to the police that Dahmer was lying and that he was using physical force against Konerak before the officers' arrival, but they were ignored. According to the police, Dahmer's behaviour suggested embarrassment. He told them that 'everybody has to be into something.' One officer later testified that Dahmer 'appeared to be a normal individual' and that they were 'convinced that all was well.' Therefore, without running Dahmer's name for warrants or arrests, the officers helped to return Konerak to Dahmer's apartment. Shortly after the police left, Dahmer proceeded to finish what he had started and murdered Konerak.

Suggesting that consensual violence is a normal part of a gay life style could arguably be the cause of more, not less, sexual orientation discrimination. The public perception of what is 'normal' behaviour in a homosexual relationship is often based on crude stereotypes of the sexual deviant. This perception is illustrated by the reaction of police officers in the case of Konerak Sinthasomphone, Jeffrey Dahmer's fourteen-year-old victim. Before Dahmer's killing spree was finally ended, the police had the opportunity to stop him and thereby save the lives of five young men. However, because the officers involved believed that violence was the norm in a male homosexual relationship, they failed to intervene, and Dahmer was free to kill again and again.

The main problem here is that the State claims a complete monopoly on violence and woe betide anybody that tries to challenge that monopoly. Courts have likened the activities of S/M defendants to acts of torture, and found that only the state is entitled to regulate activities involving the infliction of physical harm. Government trained and sponsored assassins are hailed as national heroes. Without such sanction, they are classed as murderers. The authorities use the treat of violence to make citizens comply and are therefore very unwilling to let individuals have similar powers. You might be surprised to learn for example that duelling laws were not outlawed to protect the public. Instead it was made illegal so that young men who might be needed for military service would not be able to injure and maim each other. That was after all was the prerogative of the state.

In addition, if a man is killed in what the state describes as 'sportsmanship, manly and gentlemanly behaviour,' which refers to the openly gladiatorial activities of football or boxing, his actions cannot be punished under the law. This means that you can be sent to jail for beating a consenting partner with a paddle in the privacy of your own home. If on the other hand you beat another man to death in front of thousands, maybe millions of spectators, this is gentlemanly behaviour and is exempt from punishment.

The law is intended to prevent the powerful from hurting the powerless but is that really the case? According to the San Francisco Spine Institute at Seton Medical Centre in Daly City, California, up to 1.5 million young men participate in football annually, and there are an estimated 1.2 million football-related injuries per year. In a 2010 study by Purdue University and Indiana University, an estimated 43,000 to 67,000 football players suffer a concussion every season.

However, because many injuries go unreported, the true number may exceed 100,000. The high school concussion figure is nearly double that of the next-highest sport, lacrosse.

Gridiron football, a sport where violent hitting is not just expected, but encouraged has never been more popular. A rookie's base pay next season is more than $40,000 and yet a survey of 500 retired players, fewer than half would recommend their children to play it today. Almost half of those surveyed said team doctors prioritized interests of the team over their health and eight in ten now report suffering from pain that lasts most of the day. Nine in ten players reported playing while hurt during their careers, and 56 percent said they did so "frequently." Nearly seven in ten said they felt they had no choice in doing so. "If you didn't hurt while you were playing, then you weren't playing," said one ex-professional. Team reunions usually include dinner and a golf outing. But a lot of the players are not even capable of playing golf anymore. They just go and ride around in the golf carts.

There are those whose thirst for violence remains unsated, who enjoy a 'good hit' even if it cripples a player for life, glorifying vicious, and gratuitous, contact. The violence in the Roman Colosseum increased in savagery as the Roman empire declined. If we can turn our heads toward the television and ignore the damage the players receive, what does that say about us? In both the city of Rome and Constantinople, gladiatorial contests were high priority right up until the time that the city was taken over by the invading 'barbarians' - so much so that the people in the stands were so hungry that at the end of the 'games' for the day, it was common for the people to ask 'how much for THAT meat?!!'

Although the number of boxers who have died as a result of the sport is not accurately known, it does appear that death rates are much lower than in some sports, such as horse racing for instance The American Association of Neurological Surgeons say that 90% of boxers sustain a brain injury. Boxing may account for fewer deaths than some other sports but the numbers of boxers suffering brain damage are believed to be much higher than recorded. This does not take into account the growing popularity of MMA. About one-third of professional mixed martial arts matches end in knockout or technical knockout leading to a head trauma rate that vastly out-paces football and hockey.

There are many different scenarios in which two partners can enact a master and slave fantasy, each with differing levels of physicality. In a parallel dimension, slaves might be might be conditioned to regard themselves as a certain form of specially privileged and protected citizen, necessary and loyal daughters of the great, loving mother, even though they are kept behind high, electrified fences, in lush garden surroundings. These fantasies can be elaborated in thousands of exciting permutations. The main problem for most people is that the master slave roles that are institutionalised into our own societies are those of boss and worker or ruler and citizen. Few of us have any experience as a dominant master or submissive sex slave. Here then are some pointers for those of you who might not be familiar with these fantasies.

Anticipation tends to whet the sexual appetite, as it can that for food or drink. Let us suppose that your partner wishes to be a slave girl for the evening if and only if she wears a certain set of earrings. This is an understood signal. Perhaps he has a certain ring he wears. The earrings may be understood as 'those of a slave girl,' the ring as 'that of a Master,' etc. Thus, even in the presence of a family, or relatives, or business acquaintances, etc., secretly, they communicate to one another their desires and intentions. It is another secret which they, as lovers, share. The others do not suspect.

Different women, and men, find different things sexually stimulating. Investigate one another's preferences and desires. For example, does she like, while lying bound in bed, to be fed crusts of bread, or given drink from a canteen or bottle thrust between her teeth? Does she like to be forced to eat chocolates, perhaps pretend aphrodisiacs, while she is chained and you are caressing the most intimate parts of her body? Does she like to pretend she is forced to eat from a pan on the floor, her hands bound behind her back? Does she like, lying on her stomach, a pillow stuffed between her legs, to pretend she is being beaten? Does it thrill her to respond, as a slave, to signals, such as hand clappings, snapping fingers, gestures and, even, let us suppose, whistles? Does it thrill her to drink wine from a cup which you hold for her, she perhaps bound or chained? Does it thrill her to be ordered to dance naked before you, etc.? Human beings differ very much, one from the other. Almost every human being will have a number of ideas which will seem exciting or delightful to him. Something that seems delightful to A, of course, may not seem so to B, and vice-versa.

Slaves should remember that in the context of the fantasy, he is your master. Treat him as such, literally. Remember that you are nothing; you may be bought or sold, or disposed of; you have been captured or purchased; if it pleases him, he may have you whipped or slain; fear him, he owns you; struggle to please him, knowing what may be your fate if you do not; hope that he will be kind to you; be frightened that you might not please him.

Masters should look upon their submissive as only a slave; be harsh; command her; treat her as such. In the context of the fantasy, realities are transformed. You may not even have seen this woman before the evening. Gone is your existing relationship of the past. The only reality now is the new reality. Look at her carefully, your new female slave. What will you do with her? How do you remove her clothing? Do you do it slowly and elegantly, or roughly with fervour and passion? When you unhook her brassiere letting it simply fall to the floor, or do you jerk it away, startling her? But, do you leave her her earrings? Do you wipe even the lipstick of civilization from her mouth, baring her totally to you? Do you leave her a necklace, bracelets, a slender black choker? Perhaps she is stripped with great courtesy, with gentleness and elegance, and then, by contrast, rudely ordered to the bed or floor as a captive whore. Perhaps the girl is treated with marvellous gentlemanliness and respect until the anklet or collar is fastened on her, and then, by contrast, she is harshly and brutally commanded, as the mere slave girl she now is. Shifts of treatment accorded to the woman can often be sexually stimulating to her, shaking her up and making her relate, in the context of the love fantasy, suddenly, differently to you.

Even putting on a slave garment, or costume, can be sexually stimulating to her. It can bring about a change in her fantasy personality. She stands there before you, as though furious, her fists clenched, in the garment you have commanded her to wear, that of a slave girl. If you think your girl would look well with a tiny ring in her nose, you can find an earring for girls who do not have their ears pierced, and, gently, that you not hurt her, clamp this to the sides of her septum. She must be permitted, of course, to see how she looks with such a scandalous pagan adornment. A full-length mirror in the bedroom is desirable. Women love to see how exciting and desirable they appear. If they see how marvellously they "look the part,' they will enjoy, even more, playing the part. Women are born actresses and lovers.

Remember that in all these fantasies, verbal exchanges, conversation, is extremely important. Talk is sexually stimulating, extremely so. The surest path to orgasm lies through the brain, which controls these matters. In the role of master her eyes not yet permitted to meet yours. Not until you utter the words "Please me, slave." Her eyes suddenly meet yours, for the instant defiant. Then, beneath your gaze, her eyes fall, her lip trembles. She is terrified. She, a female, has looked into the eyes of a dominant male. "Yes, Master," she whispers. See that her subjugation is complete, helpless and exacting. A slave girl must yield all to her master; she is not permitted inhibitions or reservations. Command her. Focus on her complete subjugation, her complete, deeply desired domination by an uncompromisingly triumphant male. Each woman is incomplete and partial until made whole by her surrender to a male. Some women learn love only in chains. After she has pleased you, perhaps you command her to the kitchens, or to her kennel, where a guard will see that she is chained for the night. If you are generous, however, and fond of the slave, neither bored nor irritated, you might, as an unusual privilege, permit her to remain the night in your compartments. She might be chained at the foot of your vast couch, that of the master. Or, if you wish, you may permit her to curl up, lovingly, obediently, at your side, beneath the covers. The mixture of the mental and physical is an incredible psychological alchemy, a wonder of untrammelled exoticism. The uncertainty, particularly in the case of the woman, produces a fringe of fear. Fear in a female is not at all incompatible with her sexuality. A bit of fear, and not knowing what is to be done with her, makes her more vulnerable, more submissive.

Whenever I am with a new lover and things are getting heated, I make sure to introduce a safe word. This codeword means stop, unconditionally. Often when women say "Stop" or "No" is just means "Try something else" or "Not quite yet". Only the safe word truly means stop. The codeword that I often employ is 'Red Light.' This way she can resist verbally as much as she wants, but at the back of her mind she knows she can terminate any action with the phrase 'Red Light.' This creates trust but some people prefer something more light hearted and humorous. I know of one gentlemen who uses words like aardvark and bananas because he thinks they are hilarious. Any discomfort she may feel is instantly diminished with such a stupid phrase. The codeword creates a playful dynamic to an otherwise primal act. He claims that she will be less inclined to use a funny unsexy word. Such a word would completely destroy the mood, so if she uses it you know she means business. Be aware that the same phrase can sound different under normal circumstances. When I first play with a new sub, I make them say it three times....once while pretending to be orgasmic, once while pretending to be in pain, and once while pretending to be emotionally compromised. If you plan on gagging her then you two need to set up a non-verbal mode of communicating. There should be a specific way of movement or a hand gesture to allow for her to communicate how she is feeling. There can also be a safe object. That can be held until a signal is needed, then dropped. I find that horse bells work nicely and I have heard of another couple that uses a two inch sleigh bell. When she is bound and gagged, this is where your going to have to step up as a Dominant and continuously check on her status throughout the course of the play. Hand gestures do work but you have to make sure you do not get so distracted that you do not notice. Perhaps if you cannot keep control of your urges and/or the presence of mind to pay attention to the submissive whom has charged you with their care and well being, then maybe you should be trying something a little less advanced.

Here a few interesting slave fantasies that you might like to try:

The first involves a special kind of lottery where the prize is not money but a specially selected sex slave. Citizens buy tickets as normal but the winner receives a fully trained slave rather than a cash prize. In this alternative society, the most attractive human specimens are selected randomly, and then marked and collared as a love prize. They are then given detailed and thorough training in the Venusian arts of sensuous delight. The lottery is state controlled, and its conditions are carefully regulated. The prizes must meet the highest standards in terms of health and aesthetics. This fantasy allows ample scope for a slave's feelings to be fully explored. How do they feel once selected, while undergoing training, when they are waiting handcuffed, to be won? Then there is delivery or collection. Perhaps they have been won by someone they find sexually repulsive, or perhaps it is a complete stranger. The lottery could always be of a darker more underground nature. Secretly organised by dark elements of the mafia underworld, in which tickets are high priced and are made available only to rich, screened buyers. Perhaps a student visiting a foreign country, is seized for such a purpose.

An alternative scenario is where the offspring off a once rich family is publicly auctioned to pay their accumulated debts. The unfortunate is sold to satisfy the family's creditors. On the other hand, they might, if you so wish, pass directly into the hands of a hated creditor. Perhaps he had earlier offered to cancel the outstanding debts, if the heir had accepted a proposal of marriage. Now, following lengthy court proceedings, the slave is consigned to their new owner. They are stripped. Their police handcuffs are removed and replaced by those of the new owner.

Imagine a semi-legal border casino where the rich and wealthy visit to circumvent the anti-gambling regulations of their own country.

These are commonly found all over Asia with many examples in Burma and Cambodia for example. Without the rule of law, these places can be very dangerous places. Imagine a high stakes game where a rich but reckless gambler stands as the stake. There is little thought of losing, just the kicks of the risk. To their horror, they lose. To their even greater horror, they are not permitted to buy their way free. They had counted on the fact that in the unlikely event of losing, their legal representatives can offer a thousand times the going price of any human slave, but the victor is not interested. We may further suppose that there has been much rivalry between the winner and the loser, and that they have hated and despised one another. This fantasy works very well beginning with the female in earrings and evening gown, with a card table, and an entire imagined background of onlookers, gamblers, waiters and croupiers. Perhaps, when she loses she faces her adversary, eyes flashing, demanding to know what price he wants. He draws forth a pair of handcuffs from his tuxedo, and tosses them to an attendant. "Put her in these," he tells him. Will he brand her? What will he do with his beautiful slave? How will he dress her? Where will he take her? Now, to an agony of horror, she realizes she belongs to him. What will he do with her? What will be her fate? This fantasy can be a joy for a woman to act, for, once again, there is an enormous gamut of involved emotions and responses.

For those that prefer to stay closer to home try having your slave enter the room blindfolded, hands tied behind their back. You open the door for them, "Come in, my darling." You then guide them to a place beside your chair. "Kneel here, slave, and wait for me." They kneel, resting on their heels, blindfolded, hands tied and head down. Have you ever had your lover remove your clothing with her teeth?

When it is the man's turn to take on the role of slave, an interesting variation is that of the 'militant lesbian.' She waits for him as he enters the room. If you want to put her in army fatigues, and boots that is fine. She then does with him whatever she wishes. Presumably she hates men, and wishes to degrade and humiliate them. This is useful as a female vengeance fantasy. He can play the role of some male whom the female despises with a venom, maybe someone has been contemptuous of her. She then makes him pay, a thousand times over, draining him like a semen vampire.

21. Office Fantasies

A horny boss, his sexy secretary: the erotic potential for this scene is obvious. Forced blow jobs under the desk, stolen gropes in dark corners, demanding eyes from across the room, disguised words with hidden intent. The spice in this scenario is provided by the power play. The boss is on top, so to speak, and it benefits the secretary to keep him pleased. On the other hand, the secretary has her own source of power: her feminine sex appeal. Many hotels are outfitted with a desk and other work accessories, and so it is easy to play this scene out in a hotel room and let the action progress naturally to the bed. Do not neglect the dress-up possibilities: business suits and ties for the boss and blouse, skirt, hose, garters and heels for the secretary.

The seducing the boss scenario is especially good for voyeurs and exhibitionists. The secretary, intent on seducing her boss, wears extra-sexy lingerie to work: say, a new lacy bra and panty set. As he is working, she bends over and flashes her cleavage, then her panties. Then she offers to help him relax during his hard work day with a massage. What will it take for him to finally give in? In another flavour of this scenario, the boss catches a glimpse of his secretary's skimpy G-string and determines that her too-short skirt is not work-appropriate. He must therefore insist that she take it off. Immediately, a slow, sensual striptease ensues. There is nothing quite like flinging the papers off the desk, as you sprawl your partner across the top of it, and take them! Or men, bend your ladies over it, and see how good she is at taking some 'dictation.' It is a really easy fantasy to enact at home with minimal props, and again, has the added bonus of the charge that power exchange can bring to sex. Silk neck ties can make wonderful restraints, and rulers make paddles, for those who enjoy sensation play.

Perhaps you want to elaborate upon the sexual tension between you and a co-worker, the head-butting over client management or the bickering over assignments. When you go into the conference room alone to argue it out, just the two of you, you have one of those ferocious kisses that you only see in movies. Before you know it, pens and papers are scattered across the floor and you are having sex on the table. Don't you think it would be thrilling to be pinned against the fax machine for some afternoon delight? Or perhaps in the supply room where anybody could come in for some stationary. Some people might prefer the privacy that comes with getting busy in the conference room, but there is always the elevators for the real exhibitionists among you.

Maybe you prefer to imagine boss and secretary in the middle of a secret affair rather than at the beginning. In that case, try this scenario. The secretary crouches under the boss's desk, positioning herself between his legs. She is there to provide oral service while he works but of course no-one must know that she is there. Perhaps he is attending an important video meeting or on a crucial phone call, so she must be especially quiet and discreet. How far can she push things without blowing both their covers? If you are feeling extra-daring, the 'boss' can call someone (non-work-related) for real. See how long he can keep his cool.

If you are ready for a little more physical kind of role play, then imagine that you have an extremely sexy secretary but an important aspect of her work skills is lacking. She simply cannot take dictation, or types too slowly, or messes up an important memo. After one too many mistakes, the boss takes control. She needs discipline, and that means a good spanking. She winds up over the knee of her boss as he sits in his office chair. Her skirt is hiked up, exposing her panties. Start the spanking over her panties, proceed to her bare bottom: where will the action lead you both next?

If you are looking for a male fantasy, imagine that you are an executive working on the 42nd floor of a down town office tower. It is almost midnight and you are still working late trying to finish an important project. You think that you are the only one there, when all the electricity in the building goes out. It is a complete power failure. A total blackout. Suddenly, the office door bursts open and there is your boss, her curvy silhouette outlined in the sliver of street light peeking through the window. She is usually totally in control, almost icy cool, but now she is so scared that she is shivering. She rushes over to you and wraps her arms around your neck. You do your best to comfort her, she kisses you hard and begs you to make love to her.

This is not all that far removed from reality. I can still remember a transformer being hit by lightning and blown out during a huge and violent storm. At the time I was working in a large retailer in a vast shopping mall and the blackout left the entire store in pitch darkness for nearly six hours. First of all, we had to usher the customers out and close the store. Then we all stayed late trying to save the meat, the frozen goods and all the other perishables. Many of us wandered off, because there were so many workers, and in the dark, all the managers could not keep track of everyone. The store was so huge that there was no way that anybody could have known what was happening way in the back recesses. We knew that even the hidden security cams would be down and so we took advantage of the situation. One of the supervisors had previously asked me come in when they were understaffed and this was the perfect opportunity to find out if I had really detected a sexy undercurrent to her request. We found a storage room that locked from the inside and made it a rendezvous to remember.

22. PIRATES OF THE HIGH SEAS

The myths and legends of pirates are deeply embedded into our collective conciousness. It is a theme that is rich in provocative and romantic elements. Thanks to depictions by a string of deliciously handsome actors from Errol Flynn all the way up to Johnny Depp, buccaneers are seen as strong, colourful and dangerous men, without law save that imposed by their captain. If they are caught, they are hung. Accordingly, if, in the meantime, they rape and abuse a few female captives, their penalties are none the greater.

At its most simple, you are the rapacious pirate plundering the village. She is the innocent maiden in the local town. She is at home alone, minding her own business, when you come crashing through the door. She struggles, of course, but she is helpless to resist you. Swooping down on the wench, you bodily rip her clothing from her and pin her against the wall. You hold her there by the wrists while you explain what you are going to do to her. Then, finally, you ravish her until you are thoroughly satisfied.

A much more elaborate back story is very easy to conceive. Far from land, you are aboard a merchantman bound for Shanghai. The ship has huge billowing sails and wood-plank floors that smell of wet cedar. The ship has been pursued for days; it has now finally been overtaken; there has been a brief naval skirmish, complete with cannon and splintering wood. The ship has been boarded, and taken; rough men, with cutlasses, order everybody them from their cabins harshly to the deck. The female passengers, terrified in their expensive dresses, exquisite jewellery and elegant hairdos are corralled with all the other captured booty on the main deck. Lady D'Arcy, an English noblewoman of striking beauty challenges the rough looking captain, demanding their release. She is knocked to the deck like common

126

whore. Terrified, mouth bleeding, she shrinks back among the other cowering women. Their men have been killed or wounded. The killed and the wounded, alike, are thrown overboard. Sharks prowl the lapping waves below. To the laughter of the pirates, now becoming ugly and drunk on rum, the captured sailors are forced to walk the plank.

The females are given a choice. If they are truly fine ladies, as they seem to be, or as they are pretending to be, they are to be treated with elegance and respect. They will be blindfolded, their hands will be tied behind their backs, and one by one, they will walk the plank, thence to plunge to the waiting sharks. If, on the other hand, they are not really fine ladies, and are only pretending to be such, and are truly, beneath their finery, only common whores, they need not walk the plank.

Her courage bolstered, Lady D'Arcy chooses the plank. She is, accordingly, graciously escorted to the plank. There she sees the sharks twisting below, waiting eagerly. She begins to tremble. But she is blindfolded and bound, and, with cutlass points, and long pole arms, thrust out on the plank. There she is ordered to walk. She begins to walk the plank. She does not know where its end is; it is narrow; it moves beneath her; she senses the water below; she knows the hungry sharks are waiting. She cannot free her hands; she cannot see. "Walk!" the captain commands. She steps further forward. She hesitates. "Walk!" she is commanded. "No! No! No!" she weeps. "Don't kill me! I'm a whore! Just a common whore!"

She is dragged back to the deck.

"Strip the whores." orders the captain. The women are stripped on the deck. Their jewellery is taken. Their hair is unbound. The girl's hands, she who had challenged the captain and had begun to walk the plank, remain bound. Her blindfold is removed. An hour ago she was of esteemed noble blood. To the pirates she is now just another wench and slut.

"Torch the ship," orders the captain. The taken ship is set afire. The women, naked, in cargo nets with the other treasure, are swung to the deck of the pirate ship. The ropes connecting the ships are cut, and the two ships drift apart, one burning and sinking, the other filled with the victorious pirates and their booty.

What will be the fate of the women? Will the captain reserve the proud girl to himself, or will he give her, with the others, to the crew? When he gets to his port, will he keep her, or will he sell her, with the others? We may rest assured that the girl will be well used, and will serve her masters well. Their delicate, sweet pale flesh is thus completely at the mercy of the swarthy brutes. They will be forced to serve their captors well.

The pirates are an evil looking bunch with ragged clothes and many days' growth of harsh stubble. They smell of musky sweat and cheap whisky. There is a big storm brewing, and the ship is starting to creak and rock from the wind and the waves. Lady D'Arcy is tied to the main mast. Her skirt has been ripped from her waist, and her petticoats have been carelessly discarded to one side. The dirty, hungry pirates have formed a circle around her. Their eyes are gleaming, and they crudely lick their lips as they decide who is going to have the privilege of going first. They finally decide, and the fat pirate who is first is drooling with anticipation. He gets on his knees and crawls along the deck. Slowly, he begins sniffing up her calves and thighs. His wet tongue slowly licks her outer lips and she can clearly hear him sniffing her erotic pussy fragrance. Then he slides his tongue into the fold of her lips, just licking ever so slowly. This takes her breath away and she is left wondering how a high born lady of such status could possibly respond to such a thing!

If you happen to own a boat, even a small sail boat, it can make an interesting fantasy location. Even so the tying up of a captive is probably not a very good idea when actually on the water. The risk of an emergency arising or an accident occurring, while perhaps not high, is higher than we need to take. In the safety and security of the bedroom, of course, it is a different matter completely.

The opportunities for costume play are wide and varied. A trusty bandanna makes a very versatile toy. It can serve as a gag (several different types/styles), blindfold, bandit/cowboy mask, Cinderella/

hippie head wrap, impromptu bondage for wrists and, when damp, it works great for fake chloroform It also holds scents well if it is made of cotton - a way for you to smell your girlfriend without having to carry around a pair of her worn panties. Add a bandanna to an eye patch and the theme is so clear cut that you do not really need any other items to make a very convincing costume. Cutlasses are bulky and expensive and so a small knife, preferably clenched between the teeth is more than enough to convey the idea of a threatening sea dog. We all have images in our minds of privateers from the evil, terrifying Edward Teach to a witty and charming Jack Sparrow. Of course, beyond the bearded buccaneers and peg-legged scalawags with names like Blackbeard and Barbarossa, there were also female corsairs that could be used as the basis for a wonderfully erotic female domination fantasy. These infamous she-pirates of the seven seas were even more exotic than their male counterparts.

When Lady Jeanne de Clisson's husband was charged with treason and punished with decapitation, she swore revenge on France's King Philip VI. The widow sold all of her land to buy three warships, which she dubbed her Black Fleet. These were painted black, draped with blood red sails, and crewed with merciless privateers. From 1343-1356, the Lioness of Brittany sailed the English Channel, capturing the French King's ships, cutting down his crew, and beheading with an axe any aristocrat who had the misfortune to be on board.

Jacquotte Delahaye was Caribbean pirate active in the 1650s, also known as "Back from the Dead Red" due to her bright red hair. During the Golden Age of Piracy (1650s-1730s), Anne Bonny and Mary Read disguised themselves as male pirates. Many women dressed as men during this time period, in an effort to take advantage of the many rights, privileges, and freedoms that were exclusive to men. Ching Shih was a Cantonese prostitute who married a sea captain and rose to to become one of the most powerful pirates in human history, commanding a fleet of more than 1,500 ships and 80,000 sailors, controlling much of South China Sea. In the Americas there was Sadie the Goat, named for her habit of head-butting her victims before taking their cash and

Gertrude Stubbs alias 'Gunpowder Gertie, the Pirate Queen of the Kootenays.' Piracy never really went away in the Far East. Huang P'ei-mei led more than 50,000 pirates until the end of the fifties, while 'Sister Ping' operated in the '70s, '80s and '90s until she was captured and sentenced to 35 years in prison. She is due for release in 2040.

Some of the more popular fictional female corsairs, make great fantasy inspiration. Many have seen Morgan Adams as played by actress Geena Davis from the 1995 film Cutthroat Island. My own favourite inspiration is Bêlit, Queen of the Black Coast who appeared in Robert E. Howard's Conan the Barbarian tales. Apart from jewellery, she wears only sandals and a red silk girdle. Despite her race and her lack of clothing in the tropical sun, her skin is 'ivory white'. She is described in her first appearance:

"Her white ivory limbs and the ivory globes of her breasts drove a beat of fierce passion through the Cimmerian's pulse, even in the panting fury of battle. Her rich black hair, black as a Stygian night, fell in rippling burnished clusters down her supple back. "

As a seaborne reaver she ravaged the coasts of Kush as far north as Zingara aboard her ship, the Tigress. A role playing adventure adaptation, authored by Robert Traynor for the GURPS role playing system, entitled 'Conan and the Queen of the Black Coast,' published by Steve Jackson Games in 1989 should provide plenty of ideas for anybody else with a fascination for pirate fantasies.

23. Psychiatrist and Shrink Play

Instead of doctor/nurse play, some people prefer to engage in shrink play. There need not be anything physical necessarily, but the play is often more about having the 'patient' to confess the fantasies that he or she has been too embarrassed to admit.

If you wish to take this one step further than the comfort of the psychiatrist's couch then the patient might be remanded and committed, on the basis of tests, to a remote private hospital. At first she suspects nothing. She packs her bags and travels to the remote hospital. She 'reports herself in' to the reception desk and is taken upstairs in an elevator. She notes that heavy steel doors close behind her and an evil-looking nurse escorts her to a strangely sterile, white-washed room. There is one window. It is tall, and barred. The nurse takes her bags and leaves her in the room. A few moments later the nurse returns and instructs here her to strip completely, putting the clothing, even down to her jewellery, on a table in the room. She obediently complies and, in a few moments, the nurse returns to collect the discarded the clothing. The girl is left, stark naked, in the room.

After a while two more nurses arrive. These are tall and strong, both extremely butch and undoubtedly powerful. They inspect the new arrival, frightening her with their unexpected scrutiny. Suddenly she realizes they are a pair of lecherous lesbians examining her in a very uncomfortable manner. They put her in a strait jacket, which leaves her completely exposed below the navel. She is then marched along the long cold corridors, barefoot. She passes many locked rooms until she is thrust into a hospital room, with a single bed and crisp white sheets. The lesbian orderlies sit her on the bed. She is still in the strait jacket. Then, to her horror, from the bureau, they produce chain and collar, and fasten her, by the throat, to the head of the bed. They then leave her, turning off the light, locking the large steel door from the outside.

It is at least an hour before the head psychiatrist comes to the room.

He snaps on the light and informs her that this is a high security facility and that no patient has ever escaped.

"Is this part of my treatment?" she begs. "What's wrong with me? Why are you saying these things to me?"

"Do you wish to know why you are here?" he asks.

Chained by the neck to the bed, in the strait jacket, from the waist down nude, she looks at him. "Yes," she says,

"Yes!"

"You are here," he tells her, "because I wanted you."

"You're lying!" she cries.

He puts his hand on her, intimately. "No," he tells her.

She tries to draw back, but cannot escape his hand. The collar and chain by which she is confined strikes the bars at

the back of the bed.

"You have been brought here as a sex slave," he tells her.

"No!" she whispers. She cannot escape his hand. "Please, stop!" she begs.

"There are many hospitals such as these," he informs her, "Where we keep women for pleasure."

She twists her head to one side.

"You will be trained," he says, "to give exquisite pleasure to men."

"No!" she cries.

"Did you see the sadistic lesbian nurses?" he asks.

"I did ," she replies.

"Yes," he says. "Do you wish me to give you to them?"

"No! No!" she cries.

She begins to writhe under his hand.

"Will you be good?" he asks.

"Yes, yes," she weeps, "I will be good!"

"You will be trained," he says, "to perform a number of specialist acts and to serve the senior staff of this facility."

"No," she weeps, "no!"

"I see that I must give you to the nurses," he says.

"No!" she cries. "I will be good!"

"Will you do precisely what you are told?" he asks.

"Yes," she weeps.

"Yes, what?" he asks.

"Yes—Doctor," she says.

Later, stripped, the jacket and chain removed, responding to the proper bell, and instructions, her door automatically unlocking, she takes her cup and spoon and goes down the long hallway, barefoot, to the feeding room. She passes many doors, some of them barred. Where she is seen from within, by other captive beauties, she is jeered. One beautiful blond girl, nude, holding the bars of her hospital cell, says "Stupid bitch."

Her training begins immediately. She is taught many things. For example, she is taught to kiss, to grovel, to serve drinks, and to obey the snapping of whips. When she is slow to learn, or not sufficiently pleasing, she is given for beating to the lesbian nurses. She fears them immensely. They are, generally, her guards and jailers. They hate her and treat her cruelly, because she is feminine and beautiful. It is her greatest fear that she will be given to them sexually. They have terrifying pliers and eye-wateringly long syringes. "Yes, Doctor," is now the most common phrase to come from her lips.

A pillowcase, with a hole cut for the head, and a pair of man's belts, makes a very effective 'strait jacket.' A simple white lab coat adds to the authenticity, giving the doctor an air of power and authority.

24. Public Sex and Fantasy Sex Locations

Some places make an excellent backdrop for any fantasy. Just imagine having sex inside the erotic temples of Khajuraho, on the Altar Stone of Machu Piccu or in a secret oasis in the Taklaman desert. Alfresco sex can be fabulous as long as you take a few basic precautions. A unplanned drunken quickie can lead to a great deal of unplanned complications. Here are a few tips so that you will know in advance when it is a good idea and which situations are probably best avoided. This way you can maintain the illusion of spontaneity while at the same time protecting yourself and your loved one.

Timing is one important part of the event. The other is location. It is very easy to have sex in public many times without ever be caught although the odds lengthen the more drink that is involved. One trick is to always do it at night, preferably somewhere where there is plenty of vegetation to cover your activities. Sex under the stars in a field, sounds as though it would be a uniquely romantic experience. In reality, it often results only in lots of very irritating bug bites in very sensitive places. I can remember one time being sat on a park bench with a couple of beers when we decided to give it a go. She removed her panties from under her skirt, I had my pants at the thighs and she got on top. It was amazing, but afterwards we looked around and saw a tramp sitting and staring at us from about a hundred metres away. We just raised our drinks to him and laughed it off.

In some countries there is an entire subculture devoted to exactly this kind of activity. In the UK it is known as dogging and there is a very revealing UK documentary from Channel 4 entitled 'Dogging Tales' for those wanting to learn more.

On the Plane

Joining the mile high club is a long time fantasy for many travellers but in the day of budget airlines and cattle class compartments, it is probably a lot more trouble than it is worth. Toilet cubicles are so cramped that even getting inside comfortably is going to be a problem, let alone any decent level of disrobing. Cubicles come complete with the stench of powerful disinfectants or even worse an unbreathable bog smog lingering from the previous occupant. Add unexpected turbulence to the mix and it is probably one of those things best left to the imagination,

Once or twice I have been lucky enough to meet another solo traveller aboard a quiet flight but the advice I am going to offer works just as well for a couple travelling together. In that case make sure that you book one aisle seat and one window seat and it is very unlikely that they will put anybody in-between the two of you. Alternatively, look for a flight that is less busy and move to the back of the plane where there are plenty of empty rows.

Once you find you partner's foot stroking up and down the inside leg of your trousers, then it is a good time to have a back up plan. This is your queue to order a couple of drinks along with a blanket. And while you pretend to share a movie on you laptop up top, underneath your hand is up her skirt, her knickers pushed aside, and you are gently parting her lips and slowly circling her clit with your finger. She knows that she cannot moan or react no matter how aroused she may be, or else others will become suspicious. It will therefore inevitably become your goal for the pair of you to be noticed. After bringing her close and pausing several times, you finally remove my hand, when suddenly she grabs it and squeezes her legs together and begs me for release with the look in her eyes. Now is the time to slip the blanket over her seemingly sleepy head and let her return the compliment. You can then fly the rest of the way in subdued but satisfied silence, finishing the movie with grins on your faces or falling asleep until your final destination.

The Beach

On the face of it, sex on the beach sounds hot and romantic. It is so sexy that there is even a cocktail named after it. Then again, there are also cocktails that go by the name of Duck Fart, Buzzard's Breath and Brain Haemorrhage, but I do not have the urge to try the real life versions of those. It is an incredibly popular motif in film and books, lying out on the sand under the stars while the waves crash behind you.

There are two main problems regarding beach sex that are not usually mentioned. Firstly, many couples find out the hard way that in the throes of passion, you are very likely to end up with sand in literally every orifice you can imagine. This means that you will quickly discover what it feels like to exfoliate areas of your body that do not need to be exfoliated. Rug burn is nothing compared to nature's number one chafe maker. A towel will cut down on this but will never prevent the problem completely.

The second problem is the sorry state of most public beaches. If you are thinking of engaging in a little briny coitus on a popular public beach during the nocturnal hours when it is otherwise deserted, be warned that more and more beaches are being shut down every year due to high bacteria levels in the water. The latest research shows that beach sand is a very efficient filter and accumulator which collects large amounts of bacteria with the ebb and flow of tides. Unless you are in a remote part of the Andamans or Tristan Da Cunha, then there is always the chance of contracting something nasty by grinding away all nude and lascivious on the sand. In the more built up parts of the world this could lead to anything from typhoid fever, to hepatitis A and dysentery.

The Pool

If you are too drunk to make it down to the beach or too fearful of an incident involving jellyfish, then there is always the thrill of sex in the swimming pool. Just make sure you are selective about the pool you choose. Kiddy pools might look attractive but think carefully about the levels of chlorine and urine in such places. Public pools are not much better. A far wiser choice would be a private resort pool or perhaps a pool inside an upmarket apartment complex. During my younger days as a nightclub rake in Asia, I would often choose a pool over my own apartment for a one night stand. Not only was there much less resistance in persuading a girl that I had just met fifteen minutes ago to go for a swim than come back to my apartment, but it also avoided the uncomfortable awakening the following morning. In each city that I resided, I always had one pool that I choose for such encounters. Each one was inside a apartment complex popular with western multi-national expats and was usually way beyond my own budget. Even so, whenever I would show up in the wee hours of the morning, my white face guaranteed that I was never even questioned by security. In Hong Kong especially it was a real relief to have a midnight dip after working up a sweat in one of Central's nightspots. Some people will tell you that chlorinated pools create lubrication problems that can lead to 'micro-tears' and the increased possibility of infection. I never experienced this when I was younger but I would certainly be more careful now that I am older and more prone to chafing.

The Car

Back in the 50s, the practise of heading up to Make-Out Point to christen some luxurious leather upholstery seemed to be much more commonplace. Over time this parked sex seems to changed to sex while driving, perhaps because it is more thrilling? Probably not for the numerous people who have been in accidents while having sex in the car. While the idea of car sex may be kind of hot, when you factor in the intense insanity of being horribly distracted in a fast moving chunk of metal and flammable liquids, it loses a bit of its appeal. A close friend of mine told me about his own unpleasant experience. On a cross country trip with his girlfriend, he was driving and she was bored. She reached for his belt, kissing his neck, and reached into his trousers. She kissed her way down slowly and started giving some amazing head. He slouched down a little to give her lap space. She took off her shirt so her boobs could brush his legs. It was an amazing sensation and he orgasmed intensely, deep into her mouth. He was so totally focused on her that he did not how fast he was going and how slow the car in front was travelling. He slammed on the brakes and the girlfriend bumps the stick shift, throwing the car out of gear. The car behind was keeping pace with him (might even have been watching) and was definitely not ready to stop. He hit the accelerator to avoid being rear ended but it was too late. The car behind smacked into his, and his girlfriend cracked her head on the radio, spitting the contents of her mouth all over his lap. No serious injuries except for a pinched sciatic nerve from slouching but still the most awkward and embarrassing emergency room visit ever.

My advice is that driving is dangerous enough as it is, so save your sexual exploits solely for parked vehicles. Make sure that there is enough space, although trying to attain some leverage in mini or a smart car has a thrill of its own. Personally I prefer a soft-top Thunderbird with bench seats. Even more prudent advice is to park in a secluded spot where you are unlikely to be disturbed. I once made the mistake of pulling into a deserted parking lot and going to town without paying serious attentions to the surroundings. Within just fifteen minutes there was a policeman tapping on the window. What I did not realise was that I had chosen a bank parking lot to park in. Apparently a random car in the middle of the night at a bank is quite suspicious.

Nightclubs

With so many hot young things dressed in surprisingly short skirts, all pulsating and gyrating, it is hardly surprising that the adventurous amongst us may be tempted by a taste of forbidden nightclub nookie. Sneak into the bathroom with a sweaty stranger, pick a stall and go to town. Unfortunately this is the same stall where a nightclub full of tanked up clubbers have been visiting all night, most of them way to drunk to even think about aiming. The sad thing is that the ladies are not usually much better.

Taxi Cabs

Be warned that there are a number of internet sites such as taxicams. com. Cabbies have been caught in the past for having hidden cameras in the their cars to film couples in the back and, as so many girls-gone-wild have learned, what seems like a good idea at the time turns into an especially idiotic idea in retrospect. Especially when one of your workmates shares the URL of a YouTube video featuring your hairy arse and a drunken encounter, who in the cold light of day looks like a syphilitic swamp donkey. There are certainly better ways to gain your fifteen minutes of fame.

The Pursuit

The best solution to all of these downsides is to have a fantasy where the pursuit is outdoors, but the main event is in a place of relative safety. To this end I like to set up a nightmarish situation, where I pursue my partner among crowds, which do not appear to notice her. She cannot attract anybody's attention. Even policemen do not seem to hear her, or notice her. Even if someone does notice her, they are not interested in listening to her or helping her. They turn away continuing on their own business. Unshakeably, I pursue her, nearing her, following her, coming ever closer. I follow her on subways, through streets, even into buildings. She flees, ever more helpless, more terrified. At last, in a very public place, where many people pass to and fro, I apprehend her. She is caught. She screams, she struggles, but no one seems to hear her. No one pays her attention. This usually occurs in a large train station in a heavily populated metropolitan area, where she is stripped, thrown across luggage, and forcibly taken.

The majority of the chase is reality, and we invariably finish off at a large busy train station simply because it is so public. These places always have hotels nearby, and so I chase her into one of these, into which we have checked into earlier when setting up this fantasy. She flees to the safety of her room but I burst in and take her not on the bed but on a pile of luggage on the floor. In the past I have used a busy train station soundtrack to add aural effects, and I always leave curtains drawn and lights on. This gives her the female thrill of being game, and me the male thrill of being the hunter. She is, fleeing, walking swiftly, etc., in the crowds, unable to elude me. In the fantasy, we sometimes imagine not that individuals, unnoticing, pass us; but that a sizeable crowd gathers, interested, perhaps amused, to watch her helpless struggles. Her forcible seduction, at the conclusion of which she yields helplessly, a naked, conquered female, is completely public.

The analysis of such a fantasy is quite interesting if rather complex. The situation is fantastic, and, in actuality, the woman would, in a civilized situation, be amply protected. The fantasy thus has something of the pleasure of a horror movie. Wouldn't it be horrible if it were happening, but you know very well it is not really happening. This sort of comprehension can produce pleasure. There is the thrill of excitement, but, too, the knowledge that there is no real danger. Many of us love watching horror movies but that does not mean we want to be stalked by a serial killer in real life. It is the fantasy rather than the reality that is exciting. Perhaps, even, a sense of relief, that there is no actual danger, contributes its part to the pleasure. The entire situation, because of its unusual nature, has the stimulation of wildness, implausibility and novelty. It also has built into it a unique, almost dreamlike mode of female helplessness, being completely at the mercy of an attacker while theoretically in the midst of competent, immediately present defenders. There is a literary value of paradox and irony here. How helpless can one be? Feigned helplessness can be very sexually stimulating to a female. There is also in this fantasy, of course, aside from obvious elements like pursuit, capture and rape, the fantasy of public sex. The woman is publicly exposed as being beautiful, desirable and sexually vital. Her orgasm is induced publicly, before a crowd. She can no longer keep her sexual responsiveness a hidden secret. All the world now knows that she is an intensely vital, wildly sexually responsive female. Her extreme desirability has been publicly exhibited. This appeals to the narcissist in her.

The Quickie

Quickies are often thought of as the preserve of shifty office managers having affairs with their secretaries. But the sex they provide can be especially exciting if you are in a long-term relationship where spontaneous sex is just a distant memory. You are in the kitchen or hallway, or maybe in the garden. You know friends or relatives are due to knock on the door at any moment. Or you could even be out walking in the country or at the seaside, or in a bar or art gallery. You look at your partner and know that if you do not have sex that very moment, you will explode. You kiss passionately and hungrily. Your hands roam over and under clothes, but you know you can not undress – someone might surprise you at any moment. And anyway, you are in far too much of a hurry. You push your partner up against a convenient wall or seat and undo zips and buttons and pull clothes up, down and aside just enough to allow penetration. With one eye peeled to make sure you will not be caught out, you have fast and furious sex. A good position for quickie sex is to have her standing with one foot resting on a chair (or similar object) and to enter her from behind, leaving your hands free to unbutton her blouse and play with her breasts. To really enjoy a quickie you need to get the adrenaline rush that only the risk of getting caught provides. Doing it ten minutes before her mother arrives for Sunday lunch should do the trick. Or try doing it by your bedroom window in broad daylight (but do not quote me if a passing policeman wants a word).

At one time I was very lucky to have a girlfriend that enjoyed it anywhere and everywhere. Where I lead, she followed and there was hardly ever any hesitation. Sex in a public restroom, sex in the woods, sex in a changing stall at the swimming pool (that one was her idea). One time we even stripped naked in a public park and got down in the dirt. Locations and especially locations in public can really spice things up. Initially I never thought that I would do something like that and in fact I always thought that it was not worth the trouble. Silly me. I think it is key that the guy needs to be OK with potentially getting caught. You have to find the humour in that and then she will. Take her to popular but not-so-crowded tourist spots especially during the off season. Think of places like the cliffs overlooking Sydney Opera House. While car parks have already mentioned, having her suck you in a dark and deserted alleyway is always a thrill, especially if you cum on her face in public and treat her like a dirty slut. A semi-deserted parking lot works well too and there is the added advantage of having an immediate getaway if needed.

Camping

If you prefer your outdoors location to be a little more remote then I can assure you that camping sex is some of the hottest sex you can have and one of the very best parts of camping as a pastime. One advantage is simply that you are relaxed enough to actually think about sex. You are spending quality time together day in and day out. If you have kids this is even more so as many wives enjoy watching their husbands do the daddy thing which can be incredibly sexy. Usually you can set up your site so that you have optimal privacy around the fire and so making love under the stars with a roaring fire next to you is a very real option. It is amazingly romantic. You can park your vehicle, set up your tent and run a clothes line (with towels "drying" on it when you want to make love) all in certain ways to minimize the likelihood of other campers seeing you. A nice position is woman on top with your man sitting in a comfy camping chair. Something your husband may be pleasantly surprised by is that if he is leaning back while you are in reverse cowgirl position, when you move up and down on him he is going to see peaks of the fire as you thrust. It is a unique visual you may not always have access to, but you can burn it in his memory. If he is aroused by seeing you masturbate you might also try sitting on the other side of the fire from him and giving him a show. It is very exciting to do something that is a normal part of your sex life in a new way, like outside by a fire. Then there is the whole aspect of having sex in a tent or RV, depending on the kind of camping you do, that is enough to add in that spicy ingredient of variety to your sex life. Be sure you have a large, comfortable, inflatable bed if you are tenting. It is not at all enjoyable to have a rock impale your back while you are in the throws of passion. Also, have enough sleeping bags or blankets so that you are warm enough.

If you would like to try this out for yourself, there is one book that I cannot recommend enough. It is called Sex in a Tent: A Wild Couple's Guide to Getting Naughty in Nature by Michelle Waitzman. It covers amusing things like how to create a romantic dinner in a ziploc bag and how to have sex in a tent without destroying it, as well as truly helpful information like which are the most romantic camp sites in North America and how to convince a reluctant spouse. This book is not just about sex but certainly does not shy away from it either. It is far more about getting a reluctant partner out camping and hiking and then how to improve the odds of having romantic interludes. After that, it tells you how to plan a trip, how to get along while you are out there, how to keep clean, how to have romantic dinners and then tells you all the lovely ways of making sex possible that are only available outdoors. There is an entire chapter on having sex in a canoe and the story about toasting marshmallows on an open fire is so sexy that you will read it over and over again. On top of this, there are useful information sections with recipes, romantic locations and an extensive list of online resources. Camping sex is indeed one of the most fun sexual experiences that you can experience. It never fails to disappoint.

25. RAPE FANTASIES

Admittedly controversial, rape fantasy is more than a little politically incorrect. Even so, it is a very common female sexual fantasy. The vast majority of rape erotica on Amazon is bought and read by women. A 1974 study by Hariton and Singer found that being 'overpowered or forced to surrender' was the second most frequent fantasy in their survey; a 1984 study by Knafo and Jaffe ranked being overpowered as their study's most common fantasy during intercourse; and a 1988 study by Pelletier and Herold found that over half of their female respondents had fantasies of forced sex. In a 2009 study published in the Journal of Sex Research that evaluated female undergraduates at the University of North Texas, 62 percent of the women admitted to having rape fantasies, and 91 percent of those said their fantasies were either wholly or partially 'erotic.' Even in a mainstream movie like When Harry Met Sally, Sally told Harry that she dreamed of a 'faceless guy' ripping off her ever-altering clothes. The most frequently cited hypothesis for why women fantasize about being forced and coerced is that the fantasy avoids socially induced guilt—the woman does not have to admit responsibility for her sexual desires and behaviour. A 1978 study found that women with high levels of sex guilt were more likely to report fantasy themed around being overpowered, dominated, and helpless. Even so, women who report forced sex fantasies have a more positive attitude towards sexuality, contradicting the guilt hypothesis. Like with most psychological phenomena, there is no direct explanation for why some women are turned on by the notion of force while others are aroused by the idea of making love in a field of wild flowers. Some experts believe if you peel back the layers, it is related to childhood experiences of being reprimanded or controlled or overpowered. Early, primitive feelings of aggression are often wrapped up with libido. Some women explain that when growing up, their parents really made them feel like their emotions made them unlovable. The rape fantasy appeals to them because it is the same as somebody being angry or unhappy with them but still paying a great deal of attention.

Rape fantasy is actually a 'ravishment' fantasy. Rape is a violation and no one wants to be violated, but the idea of being powerless - and thus 'blameless' - is exciting to some. You can remain the virginal sweet girl while still getting to enjoy horribly awesome sex. You do not feel guilty because, "hey, he 'forced' me, teehee." Being raped in fantasy is a convenient way of getting past the big NO to sex that had been imprinted on a woman's mind since early childhood. In a rape fantasy, a woman can freely enjoy sexual pleasure without feeling guilty or inhibited. Because she is forced by the rapist or insatiable man, she does not have to feel any shame about being wantonly sexually responsive, about being a slut who really enjoys it. The fact that he ravishes her so deeply the whore deep down comes out and she can have no-holds barred dirty passionate sex. Forced sex takes all the responsibility off her shoulders.

Some argue that the rape fantasy reflects the desire, not to be raped, but to be irresistibly attractive, so attractive that the man can not resist. The rape fantasy does vary on the spectrum from being violently raped by a powerful stranger who treats her with utter indifference on the one end, to being taken by a familiar or past lover who is so in lust with her that he just can not hold himself back and he ravishes her. In almost a savage lust he sweeps her off her feet, carries her off to the bed, and ravages and has his way with her. It is an affair of pure pleasure, an exciting brush with danger. It remains an abiding female fantasy to meet a man who gives totally of himself, who lives for her, even if only for a single night of passion. In the ravished role, the fantasy is more of a 'friendly rape' Usually it is with a man she already knows or even loves, with a connection that feels special, even spiritual. Rather than violent forced sex, it is really more akin to forceful, passionate lovemaking. This fantasy does not mean that she has actually been abused or raped. The primary appeal for women, is the concept that 'someone would take them at all costs—the idea that

'I'm so unbelievably desirable that he just loses his mind."

For both men and woman, 'rape' fantasies are very common. For the man, he fantasizes about stalking and capturing a woman, finally raping her once she has been taken. For the woman, she fantasizes about being stalked and captured, finally ending with a forceful taking. Some consider these fantasies to be remnants from our evolutionary past, part of our genetic heritage. In general, when we hear the term 'rape' it comes with harsh connotations. True rape is an abhorrent act, brutal, violent act and unacceptable for any rational being. But, the fantasy use of this term often differs from its most common usage. Sometimes it refers to a desirable taking. Its intent is not to harm but to please. In the context of fantasy we do not want anyone to be injured. We envision a fantasy rape, one devoid of the brutality of the actuality. In a fantasy love rape, the intent is not to intimidate or injure. It must be delicious for both; otherwise it is pointless.

Non-consensual sex has a more prominent and accepted role in Asian and especially Japanese erotic culture than in the West. There are various artefacts that suggest this, including film, pornography, anime, computer games. In fact, I would not be surprised to see rape-themed noodles, curry cubes or even breakfast cereals. In Japan it is open to scrutiny because there is such a permissive porn industry. In other countries such as China, Indonesia and Malaysia, it is just as common a fantasy, but because there are so many Orwellian restrictions on sexual activity, it is never openly discussed.

Many men are taught that it is so wrong to force yourself on a woman, that they have mixed emotions when a woman actually asks them to do this. Rape play is some of most edgy erotic play of all but it is a hot game for those who dare to be dangerous. Pretending to rape a woman in order to get her off is a far cry from actually raping her. The difference between a rape fantasy and an actual rape is the difference between a bungee jump and being thrown off a bridge to your death. You want the adrenaline without the danger. The sweet taste of consensual forced sex fantasies is probably so much more delicious because it is such a taboo subject.

Even so, our complex societies send a lot of mixed messages to the modern man. He is told that he should be in touch with his sensitive side and then at the same time he is told that it is bad boys and alpha males that get all the hottest girls. This is especially true with the rise of the manosphere and the seduction community. Books like The Game and Mandarin Optional have generated an enormous pick-up industry that preaches male-dominance and cave-manning. This kind of male posturing may not be scientifically proven but it generates huge sums of money for the so-called pick-up gurus involved and can therefore be very influential.

I would like to tell you about two opposite ends of the spectrum. I had a friend called Darren, a stay-at-home dad, who began regularly acting out these scenarios with his wife. One night she told him that she wanted him to go further, so he grabbed her and pinned her down. "She was pretty much fighting me tooth and nail by this time." In the process, Darren found that he had tapped into memories of being molested by a couple when he was just twelve years old. "I really lost it. A lot of anger and bitterness and rage came up," he says. "And it actually really turned me on to get in touch with that rage. I soon became dependent on it: Now I can't keep it up for regular sex." His wife "got completely freaked out by what happened—we didn't even talk to each other for a few days afterwards," and their sex life has dropped off precipitously.

I have another friend called Rolli who is a very unassuming, shy young man. He finds it hard to be assertive and is regularly pushed around by bossy women. He ended up marrying a particularly unstable Chinese girl who would beat him senseless on a regular basis. He was too afraid to get a divorce, as the shame of admitting to being a beaten husband in court was simply too much for him to bear. On one occasion they they were walking down Oxford Street with his wife when she unexpectedly lost her temper and started slapping and hitting him. She gave him a really vicious kick in the balls which immediately dropped him straight to the pavement. Two passing policemen came running up and immediately arrested Rolli. "I am nearly six foot, while she is only five foot four," he later told me. "Whenever a copper sees a small Chinese girl in tears, they always immediately assume that she is the victim." He later told me that he would never act out a rape fantasy for fear of getting seriously hurt. He was completely amazed by all the women who have confided in me a desire to be dominated. In college he managed to absorb a completely incorrect view of women's sexuality: he thought women hated all forms of male dominance because it was responsible for millennia of repression and virtually all of the world's current violence and sexual exploitation. The idea that male dominance could be hot to women was totally foreign to an art-college-enrolled 20-year-old. He told me that he had tried talking dirty to a girl during sex who practically insisted, despite the fact he was extremely uncomfortable with it. He proceeded to talk dirty and ended up triggering traumatic sexual abuse memories from her childhood. It was the only time he had ever seen her cry and he said that he had never felt so disgusting in his life. Some guys just never get a break.

Regardless of what gives it allure, the rape fantasy is a powder keg of sexual politics. There has recently been a spate of cases where on line pressure groups have hounded men who were made the mistake of mentioning rape in the public sphere. Common sense dictates that you always consider worst-case scenarios when deciding whether or not to duct-tape a woman's mouth shut as she begs you to stop. You could always end up in cuffs by following your girlfriend's directions to break into her house and hold her down during rough sex and it would be very difficult to explain. Any man that talks about rape fantasies runs the risk of being publicly crucified by militant feminists. Some would say that this actually represents hypocritical double standards. Murder fantasies are quite acceptable, with brutal killing scenes being common in mainstream movies and television. Battlefield violence, mass killing and casual homicide are all common features of modern video games. In my part of the world it is very common to see little boys running around with toy guns, pretending to shoot people. What would be the reaction if a toy company released a rapist's play set with a knife, a balaclava and a bottle of chloroform? Dress up in a

Nazi uniform and pretend to kill Allied soldiers in a Hollywood movie and you might get an Oscar, but put on a swastika at an orgy and there could well be outrage. If a sexy woman in a skin-tight cat-suit slaughters people in The Avengers that is perfectly acceptable, but put that same fetishized death or violence in the context of porn flick and suddenly it is dark, evil and possibly criminal.

In criminal law, rape is an assault by a person involving sexual intercourse with another person without that person's consent. Before you know it, you have just made the sexual offenders list. I for one would certainly not like to explain to a judge that it was just a 'role-play raping' and I am sure a great many men think this way. The above scenario might be a little extreme, but it raises some good questions: Where does token resistance end? Where does one draw the line? Not every man is the 'typical' alpha male. Some guys are plain vanilla and not into any kind of kinky stuff. Even so, they do know how incriminating this kind of behaviour can appear to the outside observer. Sometimes the only difference there between rough role play and twenty years in prison is the woman not deciding she hates your guts. If this kind of play freaks you out then remember you have just as much right to say no as a woman does. Men are simply not educated about their right to draw the line. You can always say, 'Let's go carefully' or just plain 'No.' Now men who understand that no means no just have to hope that women do too. It is crucial that couples establish boundaries and agree on safe words before attempting to re-create a rape fantasy. I like to talk about it over text or email first so that I have a written record just in case.

If you are potential ravishee, then here are few guidelines for you so that you can safely act out your fantasies. What exactly is your fantasy and why do you want to act it out? Think about these questions and how you will explain this to your partner. If you do not have a partner yet, take extra care in picking someone. What do you know about this person? Do you feel comfortable with them? Today's picky avoids tomorrow's icky. How comfortable is this person with you and your fantasy? Are they as concerned for your well-being and pleasure as their own? Always ask yourselves "What if this or that goes wrong?" Then figure out how best to avoid potential pitfalls. Do not just talk it over before, but afterwards, too. A ravishing scene is a very intense experience, and it is important to help each other process your feelings and experiences.

Some people think that the best way to explore any possible interest is simply to to take the oblique, experimental approach of gently escalating bedroom activities. Some men feel that if she is into the rape scene, she will play along each step of the way and may even advance the process her self. If she is not, you will get a rebuff at some point and can apologize with plausible denial. I personally think that this approach is just asking for trouble. A much better option would be to broach the subject in conversation outside of the bedroom, when there is no suggestion of imminent sexual activity. And by broaching the subject, I mean the frank and open discussion of one's interest in rape fantasy. Discussing it as a theoretical subject, rather than proposing it as practice to be immediately implemented, would allow for the detached examination of the fantasy by both parties. The likelihood of there being a perceived threat would be greatly diminished and the pressure of coming to a quick decision would be removed. Of course, this approach also serves to illuminate for us the strength and health of our relationship in general. If there is not sufficient trust and security between us to make such a discussion possible, then the relationship may well require a more serious appraisal.

Women really want to know what you like. Unless you are with a prude or someone very shy, any woman you are involved with sexually would not have a problem with you saying something like, "Um...could I tell you a kinky little secret about me?" And ask for her kinky little secrets too. Now, I would not suggest blurting out, "I have fantasies about rape!" because the word is enough to scare many woman. If you said, "I'd really love to hold you down or tie you up and have my way with you," you are probably going to be rewarded with moist panties. Unless she is completely repulsed by the idea, go on and let her know what else you would like to do with her. "I want to rip your clothes off and slam into you while you struggle under me." Sometimes—it is all in how you phrase it. Ask her if she can wear an old dress she did not care about and allow you to rip it off her. For a lot of women the tearing of clothing has to do with urgency and not force - hence the notion of the entirely consensual 'bodice-ripper' romance. It is a distinction one has to be cautious about. Why not buy some cheap clothing from a thrift store that can be torn, sliced, or cut. Cheap, disposable clothing can lend a fun air of realism to the scenario.

Many of these fantasies concern a contest of wills, especially for a woman who is accustomed to winning but wishes to lose to this one man. He is usually powerful, strong, and arrogant. It is important for couples to discuss what her reaction will be. Some women want to be strong, just not quite as strong as he. They have to be seduced or even forced, but she always wants him, even though she may feign disgust, hatred, or indifference. A lot these fantasies are 'Taming of the Shrew' scenarios, where she is such a wild-tempered bitch that the man decides to do the impossible: to conquer her, and make her submit to him. After kissing, cuddling and necking for awhile, she might suddenly refuse to go farther. Decide in advance where she will slap and hit in the middle of a clinch. No matter how hard she fights, kicking and screaming, her clothes are ultimately ripped off her body. She wants to slapped around and fucked really hard. She wants him to call her a 'stupid whore!' and a 'filthy bitch!' Some women want a man who will pounce on her. I knew a girl who with beaming eyes confessed she wanted to be raped in a dark and lonely forest.

It does not have to be whips and chains. Some definitely prefer the more 'mental' side of it. She wants to feel helpless, used and worthless. If as a man you can learn basics of grappling then she she can fight you as hard as she can while you take her. Martial arts such as Judo and Taijitsu teach leverage points that you can use to restrain her and make her feel powerless. It is also useful to always carry some lube with you. This way you can throw her to the ground at night somewhere outdoors and act out a rape fantasy without her needing to get her wet.

151

Being raped or ravished is the fantasy that nearly all women have but most are too embarrassed to admit to. As a young man, I thought that being tender and loving was the key. They do want that too but 99% of the time they want to be taken and fucked. The key is to love your women but fuck them into submission at the same time and they will come and come again.

Nothing gets a woman hotter than her man being extremely aggressive and controlling. The first time you slap her she will likely be overwhelmed by how turned on she becomes. Women like gentle sex every now and then, but many get much more excited when they are slapped, choked and spanked. Lightly squeeze her neck for a few seconds, just enough for her to feel an increased blood pressure in the head and alter her sensations a bit, but while also allowing breathing normally. Secretly they want to have their hair pulled, get face-fucked until they gag and thrown around like a rag doll. They want to have some really wild, animalistic sex. As long as it has been agreed in advance, then do not be afraid to shove her down and fuck here brutally. Make her submit. Command her. Scratch her, bite her, break the skin. Slap her face with your dick and fuck her so hard it hurts. Make her hurt when it is over. Ensure that she will barely be able to walk for days.

Some women have probably imagined every rape scenario possible. They are often really detailed and can even become quite violent. These can include gang rape, DP, held hostage, kidnapped, date rape. The only theme that holds true throughout is it being extremely personal with plenty of forced kissing and close manhandling. Once you have ascertained that she harbours these fantasies then burst into her room and roughly grab her by the mane. Handcuff her, beat her with your belt and assault her verbally while you make her do whatever demeaning sexual act you see fit. Spit on her, emotionally abuse her and call her a whore. Make her hit you. I saw stars once when she clocked me so hard that I was the one that ended up with a black eye. Afterwards she will likely tell you that it was the best sex she has ever had. If you are very secure about yourself and your relationship it will really add to the passion but I do see how if there are any doubts about your relationship it would cause some major problems. This is why I I say that you must discuss it in advance. It really depends on the individuals but if you can pull it off it will get intense and heat things up to the max.

It does not seem to be just women, either. Plenty of men seem to be into occasional submissiveness, which is two sides of a same coin, I think. We like giving up control and power, becoming 'blameless' and completely at someone else's whim. If anything, it probably goes back to that comforting feeling of being a child, powerless and without responsibility. We have so much on our plates as adults, sometimes it can be great to just give it all up.

Rape Misadventures

Rape fantasies can be some of the most fulfilling sexual experiences that you will ever have. There is of course plenty of opportunity for things to go wrong. I will take this opportunity to share with you some of my own rape fantasy misadventures so that you can avoid similar situations.

I never used to be into the rape fantasy but living in Asia, nearly every girl I dated had this fantasy. The ones that live in conservative Asian countries often end up acting like sexually repressed Catholic schoolgirls. Having been bought up in the West where men are supposed to be thoughtful caring gentlemen, I was rather shocked when the first one asked to be raped. I think that she had done it before because she taught me about safe words and told me in great detail how she wanted to be abused. I could not believe how turned on she was and then half way through she let out the most almighty scream. Suddenly there was blood everywhere. Thick and mucus-y, with squirts of red juice dripping out all over the place. I later found out that she had become so excited that she had popped a cyst. It was not a promising start for me. I felt like I just raped and murdered Bambi.

Thanks to my geographical location, (I was still living with my family in Hong Kong) it was not long before another girlfriend started telling me about her secret fantasy. We will call her 'Amy' mostly because that's her real name. She had always been much more 'responsive' during the middle of the night and she dreamed of a guy breaking into her room after she had fallen asleep, and physically forcing himself onto her. She was very detailed in how she wanted it done. She wanted me to surprise her, literally pin her arms down with one hand, take off her top with another. I would unzip, leaving my pants on. Her panties would be kept on while being wedged to the side. Finally, I would enter her. All the while, she would be saying "no," and begging me to stop. She got incredibly horny just telling me about it. I was just starting to see a pattern emerge.

As the hour approached, I walked down to Amy's place, waving at the the guard in the security box. If only he had known my plans. I had been for late night takeaway and finished by swooshing some water in my mouth, and popping in a mint. In hindsight, maybe I was not active enough in getting into the role. I am not sure that real rapists pay so much attention to personal hygiene. My heart was already thumping by this time, and my late-night snack was starting to repeat on me. I was sweating like a... well, like a rapist. At least that part was authentic. I remember thinking that I should have worn shorts but it was too late to back out now. As soon as I got to the front door I set off the automatic lights! Good thing her bedroom did not face the road. I put the key that she had given me in the lock, and opened the door as softly as I could. The door was reasonably oiled, but still gave a slight creak. I tip-toed toward her room, and opened the door, at which point, I heard some faint tossing and turning from her parents bedroom. It felt like I stood there for a whole ten minutes, breaking out in a cold sweat. Eventually I plucked up the courage to inch towards her bed, trying to be careful not to step on anything. Realizing that my jeans would just get in the way, I slipped them off as quietly as I could. Fortunately she was quite a heavy sleeper.

As usual, she had kicked off the duvet which allowed for easy access. It was a fantastic sight. She was wearing a t-shirt jammies and boy shorts. Her long, smooth, tight, slender legs glistened in the moonlight and I just stood there for a moment, admiring the view. Then I remembered that I was here to fantasy-rape her.

I climbed slowly onto the bed, knee first on one side, and then straddling her. She was on sleeping her side and so I forcefully turned her on her back by pushing down on her right shoulder. She opened her eyes, breathed in quickly, and gasped. Actually I am not sure who panicked more. I thought that she was going to scream and I pressed my palm over her mouth. Instinctively I began whisper-shouting "Shhh shhhhhhh it's me!" It was certainly not the kind of character acting that was going to earn me an Oscar, but I was scared and I did not know what else to do. Midnight raping was not on the syllabus at my school. It might have been something that was taught to teenage Viking marauders and young barbarian Huns but at the Queen Elizabeth comprehensive school we did English and physics and home economics instead. It took her a while to register who I was so I slowly uncovered her mouth. She let out a, "What the f.....?" and almost knocked me out cold with the worst morning breath that I have ever experienced. She was still very disoriented, so I took her hands, one at a time, and placed them above her head, holding them down. Then I tried to take her t-shirt off. It was not such an easy thing to accomplish while I had one hand pinning her arms above her head. Screw it, I made an executive decision that the top stays on after all. She was looking more than a little confused at this point. I was on my knees, leaning over her, and slid my knees toward her crotch the way she always liked. She let out a long low moan. I thought that she was supposed to be pleading 'No!!" but no matter. Her hips began to slide up and down so that she could rub herself against me, and the sensation of her tight inner thighs rubbing against my leg was really making me excited. I literally sprang out of the front of my boxers, spread open her legs, and positioned myself right at the entrance.

I was actually surprised that it had not been been more difficult. I gave here a bit of a 'paint-brushing' to get some of her juices on my tip. I could tell that she was just starting to become wet. Not quite ready, though... but maybe I could be a little rough this time, that's the point, right? Anyway, by now I was too damn horny to give it a second thought and started pumping in, a little deeper with each thrust. She let out a slight "ahhh", but I could not stop. Instead of saying "no" or "stop," she just kept on saying "fuck" or "unnnn." What the hell? That was not in the script. It was fine though, because I was quickly beginning to see the appeal of surprise-sex. I finally used both my hands to spread her arms apart, and started sucking on her neck. And then suddenly -

THE LIGHTS TURN ON

Holy fuck! - Jesus jumping jacks! I look down, only to see her turn her face toward the door, and yelp loudly. I turn around, and see her mother standing at the doorway, eyes wide open, completely speechless. She pulled me off of her, which hurt like hell as I was ripped out perpendicularly. We both frantically grabbed the blanket and covered ourselves, scurrying against the wall like some frightened animals.

Mom: What are you two doing?!

I did not have a clue what to say.

GF: Mom get out!

Mom: What are you two doing?!

Me: I'm sorry! I'm sorry!

Ex: MOM!!

Her mom begins to close the door, but manages to work in a "Be more quiet!"

By now my erection had shrivelled up to the size of pea pod. My heart was pounding, and my girlfriend was is glaring at me wide-eyed, in a "What the hell were you thinking?" way. Well, excuse me for trying to fulfil your fantasy but all could muster was a,

"I don't know. I just wanted to surprise you."

I quickly got dressed, without even having a chance to wipe myself off on the curtains, and she quickly rushed me out of the house. She was still completely freaked out the next day. Her mom didn't bring it up at all, and acted like nothing had happened. As she was walking out of the house, her mom finally dropped a, "I know you have a boyfriend now, but you need to prioritize your time a little better." What does that mean??

We talked about it afterwards, and the reality was, she never expected that I would go through with it. To her, a rape-fantasy was so unrealistic that I would never have even considered it. Even so, she appreciated the effort I put into in, and thought it was funny, minus the part about her mom freaking out. This was not really the reaction that I had been hoping for and we split up shortly afterwards.

I later met a girl, beautiful, smart and very competent in her professional field, who liked to be ridiculed and punched in the face while she was giving me oral. "Be meaner, hit me harder, really bust me in the jaw." At the time I was very much "Um....no. You are a lovely person, but I am not the kind of guy who is going to get my rocks off while abusing someone else. Sorry about whatever the self-esteem issues are that makes you want to be degraded. Thanks for the great two months of dating and crazy sex." Her next boyfriend was a complete asshole, and I do not doubt he was happy to give her what she asked for. I only I had known then what I know now. At the time, I was simply afraid and making excuses. I have mammoth salmon-grabbers and I really did not need to explain a girlfriend with a busted jaw. I really did not fancy having to take her in to the emergency department and have the admissions nurse look at me with the hate of a thousand angry suns before I could defend myself. Even if I had replied "I know what you're thinking, but really, she was asking for it," I do not think it would have been a pleasant scene.

26. RELIGIOUS RITES OF PASSAGE

Sacred sexual fantasies run the entire spiritual spectrum. Some people fantasise about having sex on an altar in a church (specifically in Italy) while listening to Depeche Mode's Song of Faith and Devotion album. Others dream about an Eros angel with wings to take them flying. Dreams of flying are often considered symbols of orgasm. You might imagine a divine threesome with you, your lawfully wedded spouse and the all-embracing presence of God or the Goddess. Your sacred sex fantasies might be influenced by a religious upbringing, the Bible, the Koran, the Tao Te Ching or other spiritual teachings that elevate the sex act to something heavenly, such that you might imagine your sexual union as a cosmic merger of two souls becoming one. Fantasies of sex with space aliens and superheroes might even fit into the "angel" category by some more open-minded types.

For most of us though it is more about priests and nuns becoming curious about their sexuality rather than heavenly beings. Some might be a bit more animal. Perhaps she can pretend she is the devil incarnate sent to tempt the holy man of God. Nuns being raped seems to be a popular theme in porn and even one that has been explored in mainstream Hollywood movies such as American Horror Story Asylum but the difficulties in obtaining an authentic nun's habit generally makes this kind of fantasy highly impractical.

The overarching attitude of the church is that sex is sinful unless you are trying to procreate. John Paul II's Theology of the Body was pro-sex-enjoyment. For the married folks, of course. Other more liberal preacher's believe that "Sex is beautiful and wonderful, and God made it to be beautiful and wonderful." Polish Priest Ksawery Knotz has even written a "Catholic Kama Sutra" telling Catholics that sex should be, "saucy, surprising and fantasy packed." Poles bought

5,000 copies of *Sex As You Don't Know It: For Married Couples Who Love God*. The tome contains explicit advice on theological and practical issues about sex, including oral sex, contraception, and the importance the wife being satisfied during sex. "Some people, when they hear about the holiness of married sex, immediately imagine that such sex has to be deprived of joy, frivolous play, fantasy and attractive positions," writes Knotz, a Franciscan friar from a monastery outside Krakow. He argues that sex is an important way for married couples to express their love and grow closer to God, and can include oral sex and manual stimulation. "Every act - a type of caress, a sexual position - with the goal of arousal is permitted and pleases God," he says. Some have questioned the monk's expertise on sex, since he is celibate, but he says he learned about sex from counselling married couples and running a website that gives sex advice for Catholics. "I look at it this way: you do not have to have a heart condition to be a cardiologist and you do not have to be an alcoholic to work as a therapist." No one should be ashamed to enjoy sex and religious folk rarely talk about how good it is for your marriage to have a great sex life. For Protestants there is a fun blog called christiannymphos.org with a similar anything goes mentality.

There are still plenty of sex fantasies that would likely make members of the church choke on the tea and biscuits. Exorcism is a complex role-playing scenario, good for psychological interplay. In this scenario, one partner is possessed by a demon; the other partner is a member of the clergy called in to cast out the evil spirit. The demon does not want to go, of course, and will do anything, up to and including trying to seduce the clergyman, to escape. Complicating the scenario is the fact that the person possessed by the demon is sexually chaste and naive, and is quite shocked by the things the demon is making him or her do; complicating it still further is the fact that the clergyman is also sexually naive and inexperienced. So the evil demon forces a sexually timid person to seduce the inexperienced priest in some extremely vulgar and profane ways, much to the chagrin of the person whose body the demon has inhabited, and is using... This

159

scenario can allow you to really play up the virgin/whore dichotomy. It also allows for a great deal of very kinky humiliation play, where the person possessed by the demon will describe himself or herself in graphic and vulgar terms, and perform very kinky actions, while still trying to 'resist' doing these things. Will the priest be able to cast out the demon before both people lose their purity? Probably not...

Another risqué setting is the young lady who confesses to her priest and must do penance.

"Enter," comes a deep voice from the darkness and she obeys, opening the door and seating herself on the narrow wooden bench, the darkness both comforting and frightening. "What may I do for you, my child?"

"I have been a bad girl, Father. I wish to confess my sins."

"Certainly. When was your last confession?"

"One week ago, Father."

"Ah, yes, I remember. You have already sinned again? Shame on you, young lady!"

"Yes, Father. I am ashamed. My sin is this: though I am but recently married, at school this week I lusted after a man."

"Oh?"

"Yes," continued the pretty girl, her face flushing despite the darkness that cloaked her. "A professor, in fact."

"This is not good, my child."

"Even worse, Father, he is married."

"Definitely forbidden!"

"I know, Father, but I cannot help it. When I am in his class all I can do is imagine us together, his arms around me, his lips kissing me, his hand touching my-"

"Enough, child! Do you want to commit yet another sin?"

"No, Father."

"Is this all you have done? Just 'think' about committing a sin?"

"Yes, Father. But I need to serve penance to remind myself to be good."

There was a long pause from the disembodied voice on the other side of the thin panel. Then the man spoke. "Are you sure, girl? Your sin is quite severe, I'm afraid. Lust and a potential extra-marital affair require substantial punishment."

"Yes, Father. Whatever you think is appropriate."

The priest clucked his tongue at this and scolded the girl.

"All right, my child. Please go to the back of the church to my office and wait for me. Here in the key."

Until I started writing about this, I had absolutely no idea that I wanted to receive head inside of a confessional box. While anything taboo is definitely a turn on, just the idea of this scenario gives me an erection so hard that it might tear through my jeans. If you have the same uncontrollable urges then here is a scenario that you might like to try. A male priest is conducting confessions and a highly promiscuous girl goes into the booth to explain how she has been having very dirty thoughts. She just cannot help but think of sex all the time and she even tries to tempt the father away for some action. When she finds out that you the priest, have given up your sexuality for priesthood, she desperately wants to take it away from you by fucking you against your will. She describes how she would tie your hands to a chair, give you the most amazing blow job and then proceed to rape you. All the time, you have to be saying things like "Stop it my child! I gave up my life for God!" In return she would be saying things like "Hmm Reverend...if you don't want to have sex, why do you have such a hard cock?" "God is watching you right now and is disgusted by how corrupt your thoughts are." or "Where is your God now?"

27. ROBOT SEX

Men and women are already having sex with robots to some degree. They are extremely crude robots. But by the strictest definitions, they robots all the same. The vibrator. The mechanical penis pump. They are both mechanical devices meant to do the work of a man... or woman. But it does not stop there.

With the advent of silicone-based sex dolls like RealDolls and SuperDolls, the idea of sex with robots becomes more and more realized. Even though they are priced between 3000 and 6000 dollars US, they are especially popular on Chinese equivalents to eBay, where much of the country suffers from a distinct shortage of real women. As prostitution increases driven by the ever increasing wealth gap, this trend is likely to continue. Completely customizable in appearance; 'dollers' are already deviating from the constraints of the traditional human design, having dolls made for themselves in colours straight out of science fiction. Scales, horns and blue skin. Female designs with penises AND vaginal openings. Even so, reducing women to a set of remote controlled tits and boobs, with three orifices, preferably tight and moist, is still a very poor second choice for most people.

The machines that we are waiting for are not sex dolls but real 'sexy robots' the alluring gynoids seen in the artwork of Japanese airbrush artist, Hajime Sorayama. Remember the most convulsive, brain-ripping climax you ever had? The one that left you with "I could die happy now" satiety? It is these kinds of orgasms, the hormone-exploding orgasms that are excellent for mental and physical health which we will eventually enjoy with carnal cyborgs. Sexbots will electrocute our flesh with climaxes far more intense than we have ever known because as partners they will be more desirable, patient, eager, and altruistic than their meat-bag competition. In addition, they will have been be uploaded with supreme sex-skills from millennia of erotic manuals, archives and academic experiments, and their anatomy will feature a huge range of specially developed sexplosive devices. Sexbots will heighten our ecstasy until we have shrieking, frothy, bug-eyed, amnesia-inducing orgasms. Look forward to quadruple-tongued cunnilingus, open-throat silky fellatio, deliriously gentle kissing, transcendent nipple tweaking, g-spot massage and prostate milking dexterity, plus 2,000 varieties of coital rhythm with scented lubes.

At the moment we are still awaiting truly sentient robots, but for many the fetish is so strong that the reality cannot be far off. Once babies are grown in test tubes, might we genetically engineer all children to be male, foolishly considering them to be the superior sex? Will robot women then be artificially manufactured for the sole purpose of being our sex toys?

For the time being there is a lively robot fetishism sub-culture which is often referred to as ASFR (i.e., alt.sex.fetish.robots, based on the name of a now defunct internet newsgroup) or technosexuality. Just as members of the furry fandom, who become sexually excited by imagining themselves transform into an animal or animal hybrid, techno-fetishists yearn for the cold, hard metal embrace of an artificial being with lifeless eyes obscured in a parody of the human love. There are similarities to mechanophilia (i.e., sexual arousal from cars or other machines and sometimes referred to as 'mechasexuality') although the specific desire is to have a ready-made android or gynoid [female robot] partner that is desired for sex and companionship. Some of these individuals like to imagine removing skin or body parts to reveal electronic circuitry becoming arouseD by anything from the Six Million Dollar Man through to The Terminator. Others are more interested in techno-transformation. This involves themselves or their partner (or even both) being either willingly or unwillingly turned into an android.

Unfortunately for these robofans, thanks to a lack of advanced technology, the real life expression of technosexuality is still somewhat limited. This is still a very large market for techno-sexual art has developed which caters for robot fetishism

Our fascination with the concept of an artificial lover dates back into ancient mythology. Pygmalion is the name of a sculptor from Greek Myth. He was aloof and cold to the women that wanted him, for none could match the beauty of the fantasy ideal he had in mind. He started eventually to sculpt from ivory the image of Aphrodite, Goddess of Love, but in doing so, fell in love with the statue and started to sculpt her into the image of his ideal woman. Moved by his efforts, Aphrodite granted the statue, Galatea (Sleeping Love), life so it could return his love. Boiled down to its very essence, the myth tells the story of a person that created the ideal lover. And of course we get the resurgence of the Pygmalion meme with movies like 'My Fair Lady' and eventually Kim Cattrall in 'Mannequin.'

In the early black and white classic 'Metropolis' the mad inventor Rotwang kidnaps the heroine Maria. He has created a robot to be a replacement for a woman he loved, but it needed a soul so he imprints the image of Maria onto his Robot. The scene itself is filled with the trappings of the mad scientist film long before Dr. Frankenstein's lab. This is a reoccurring theme with mad scientists creating robots or dolls that come to life. There is the Bride of Frankenstein but even Chitty Chitty Bang Bang, where the character of Truly Scrumptious is dressed in an Austrian Dirndl, and made up to look like a wind-up doll. Benny Hill, the toymaker, winds her up and she proceeds to perform a little song and dance number for the King of Vulgaria, after which she slows to a stop when her mainspring winds down. There are a number of pulp serials full of hypnotized femmes such as Star Trek, The Twilight Zone, and My Living Doll. We still see the Frankenstein Complex in such creations such as Westworld, The Stepford Wives, and Star Trek, but now there is an added tone of eroticism. Priss played by Darryl Hannah is even cited as 'Your Basic Pleasure Model' and the blatant sexuality Jeri Ryan playing the infamous borg, Seven-of-Nine on Star Trek Voyager is unequivocal. Even in music the subject of robot fetishism has been explored with albums such as Frank Zappa's concept LP, Joe's Garage.

While advanced sexbots remain firmly in the realms of science fiction, there is still an opportunity to experience robot sex through role-play It is easy to imagine a human looking android that can to be activated or deactivated in all sorts of ways. The hypno-slave or living mannequin clearly needs a controller and this could be a wide range of fantasy roles ; The User, Mad Scientist, Hypnotist, Sculptor, Master/ Mistress, Programmer, Gorgon, Space-Alien, etc. The controlled person might be a posable plastic or fibreglass mannequin, a tranced down living model serving as a mannequin or statue in a state of posable catalepsy (hypnotically frozen.) In the late 1970's series, Buck Rogers in the 25th Century, the hero is captured by the Draconian Princess Ardala, who copies his form and creates three android versions of him, subservient to her will. These android copies, she activates with a TV remote control-like device, which causes the still and blank-looking Buck-bots to be illuminated around the eyes for a moment and come to life. For a more technologically advanced scenario, slave-bot nanites (sub-cellular sized machines) can be implanted or worn on an attached or attached device. The methods by which technosexual themes can be applied to mind control erotica seem only limited by the imagination. Using implanted or installed technology to seduce, hypnotize and program people into robot-like positions of servitude makes for an interesting sexual fantasy. People can become the perfect servant for the one they wish to serve.

The sexual arousal may be heightened the more that the person imagined or dressed as a robot sounds and acts in a robotic-like manner. Think of the old stereotypical hypnotic fantasy, where someone might have both arms out in front of them, staring blankly ahead at nothing in particular, saying, "I.HEAR.AND.I.O.BEY.MAS.TER." Stuttering, random words or erratic speech patterns, speech slow-down or speed-up can all be indicative of malfunction. Sometimes all that is required is a monotone and clipped delivery, pausing for a brief beat between words or syllables. Do not forget the appropriate facial expression. The Blank Look. The 1000-Yard Stare. The Stoneface. Sometimes it could be silver or circuit imprinted contact lenses.

Consider the simple act of reaching for your coffee cup. Break that down into its individual parts: Turn head to orient vision on cup, Raise

Arm, Extend Arm, Extend Fingers, Rotate hand for grasping, Extend hand around cup, Close fingers around cup, Lift, and so on and so on. Breaking down movements into individual actions can seem mime-like. And some of the best examples in media can still be found in the performances of mime artists like Shields and Yarnell who were regulars on the now infamous Donny and Marie Osmond Variety Show in the 1970's. They were quite well known for their portrayal of 'The Klanks' a robotic husband and wife that moved robotically, with typically blank expressions on their faces. Later, Darlene Yarnell has been used in all sorts of robotic parts in which she moved in the same stilted mechanical fashion, most notably as the character 'Dot Matrix', voiced by Joan Rivers in the Mel Brooks movie, Spaceballs. Some good examples of robotic movement can be found at www. mannequeen.com, where you can download movies of women acting in a robotic or toy-like fashion.

Of course, technology need not always come in a humanoid form. The machine here can be can be something, through which, nude and helpless, she is processed. For best results, perhaps this machine should figure in the context of a larger fantasy. Perhaps it is used to punish a disobedient female, and its attentions, hydraulic and mechanical, are unpleasant and designed to drive her back, eagerly and submissively, into the arms of a live male. Or perhaps it is the product of a scientific misogynist, who enjoys, through observation windows, noting the distress and helpless responsiveness of a despised sex. A turnabout fantasy would be that of the politically powerful lesbian misanthrope who contrives such a machine to humiliate and rape males. Another possibility, more interesting, is that it is an advanced culture's device for removing frigidity in captive females. When the machine finishes with the woman she is not only sexually vital, sexually alive, but an incredibly powerful sexual desire, in the throes of which she often finds herself helpless, has been instilled in her. Perhaps the machine more arouses her than satisfies her. Perhaps it teaches her more what she is missing than gives it to her. Perhaps, in effect, it readies her, and superbly, for male sexual domination. It brings her to the point where her needs now cry out for satisfaction, and at the hands of a handsome, powerful male. Perhaps, when the woman comes out of the machine, she is certified, or stamped, in some way, depending on the adequacy of her responses and the registration of these by the machine. She emerges marked as 'Grade A' and packaged for shipment? There might even be an industry devoted to the capture and 'process' Earth females in this fashion for mercantile distribution throughout the galaxy, where such females might be desired, e.g., in remote Earth colonies or among more humanoid aliens, who might desire them as slaves or sex animals.

As technology expands so do our ideas surrounding technosexuality. As one writer stated 'We are all interested in the future, for that is where you and I are going to spend the rest of our lives.' It has been predicted that the arrival of 3D printing is going to drastically accelerate robot development. There is also a greater need in many twenty first century humans for alternatives to human companionship. Not only are we now conditioned to interact with machines on a daily basis but many of us are now being diagnosed with social anxiety. For aspies and those with borderline autism, an AI (or even a primitive computer of today) is perfect, calm, and predictable. It acts exactly as it was programmed to. Technofets are quickly learning what pushes their buttons and so robosex is undoubtedly going to play a major role in our future.

28. ROCK STARS AND GROUPIES

Music related fantasies can be just as a wild and outrageous as any of the most extreme S&M scenarios. Here is one from an internet poster who prefers to remain anonymous:

"One of my favourites is a dream about the Cockettes. I'm part of their show, and we're all on stage. They're bisexual, and they come out pretty naked in some far out costumes. And I run around in a black slip dressed like my mother. Everybody's grabbing cocks and tits. There's the longest possible line of people grabbing each other, somehow, up on the stage. And you know what? By the time we really get into each other, the audience is doing it too!"

Actually this sounds pretty similar to a GWAR show that I went to see at Rock City when I was teenager. I am pretty sure that anybody who went to see Iggy and the Stooges or Wendy O'Williams and the Plasmatics has similarly fond memories.

The decadent lifestyles of rock and roll stars are legendary. Just watch any rock band documentary on the Biography Channel and you will hear stories of the most loyal fans that are willing to do anything to please them – the groupies. Sex with young beautiful groupies is just one of the many perks of life as a musician on the road. Imagine that you have just rocked an entire stadium's worth of fans. You picked out the super-hot, starstruck little number in the front row and had a roadie give her a backstage pass while you played the encore. Now you and she are heading back to the hotel together for a night of partying. Order the champagne room service and some extra towels. Ask her for the most outrageous sexual favours. She is a groupie, after all, and she will always be eager to please. Show her that your fingers are talented at more things than just playing a guitar. Maybe she has a few groupie sex tricks up her sleeve she would like to try on you, too.

One of the other perks is, of course, that sweet hotel room suite. Put the two together and watch the sparks fly. Groupies should dress in their slutty best. By doing this you can often get the other hotel guests wondering who you really are, because you are obviously famous but they cannot quite place you... Once you are behind closed doors, show some courtesy to the hotel and do not really trash the room like the rock stars of old. TVs tossed into swimming pools are very last millennium. Mess up the sheets, dirty some room service dishes and a fling around a few damp towels to create the right ambiance, if you are into that sort of thing.

Sometimes groupies get carried away in their enthusiasm for their favourite star and go a little too far. Like breaking into hotel rooms. In an exciting alternative scenario, the groupie has somehow gotten access to the rock star's suite and is waiting for her opportunity to pounce. She can start by demanding an autograph on her cleavage, but that certainly will not be enough to satisfy her completely. Her demands will escalate – can she have an item of clothing as a memento of her meeting? And how will the rock star handle it if she asks for a pair of his underwear? Of course, maybe he is not even wearing any underwear. Maybe she would be willing to accept a different kind of souvenir instead.

In some ways, this role play is even hotter when it is turned upside-down and the girl gets to be the rock star, cool and in charge. Start at a nearby dive bar. Make sure that you glam it up and dress the part – dramatic make-up, lots of tight leather and plenty of attitude. The male groupie buys the star a drink from the bar. She accepts, but keeps it cold as ice. He tries to flirt with her, make some small talk and get the jukebox jumping but she does not even remove her sunglasses. If you want to get kinky, have him get down on his knees and beg for her to come back to the hotel with him. Otherwise, after she finishes her drink, she can wordlessly grab him by the collar or lapel and drag him off to her hotel hideaway for a night of being treated like a piece of meat.

29. ROLE REVERSALS

Taking on the traditionally male dominant role gives women an outlet to vent their frustrations. It helps them think better of themselves and improves their self esteem. It releases suppressed emotions and ventilates often-bottled hostility and aggression. It gives them more self-respect and helps them to be freer, happier human beings. There are pleasures in being the leader, the commander. Many of us are led to believe in the natural existence and history of hierarchical structures. We are taught to believe that there was always order and structure in human groupings, leadership by an elite of strong, dominant males, and, thence, downward through a social hierarchy. As our understand of ancient history increases this is looking less and less likely. A good place to begin is the critically acclaimed Chalice and the Blade by Rianne Eisler. The patriarchal societies that we have all come to accept as the norm may in fact only be a very recent development in human history. Books like this might be the confidence boost that some women need to express their sexuality in a much more dominant form.

Petticoating, also called pinaforing, is a type of forced feminization that involves dressing a man or boy in girls' clothing. While the practice has come to be a rare, socially unacceptable form of humiliating punishment, it has risen up as a popular sub-genre of erotic literature. Of course, cross dressing need not always create a subservient, submissive character. As a youngster I spent many a happy evening at screenings of the Rocky Horror Picture Show, outrageously dressed as the sweet transvestite Dr. Franknfurter, played in the film by Tim Curry. Despite the lipstick, the basque, the stockings and suspenders, this was a role of macho virility and confident dominance. I paraded around with a string of sexy French maid girlfriends, beating and berating bald butlers and seducing the beautiful young visitors. An important precursor to the rapidly expanding cosplay movement, Rocky Horror has long been an opportunity to make an exploratory foray into the world of kink parties and sexual deviance. Rocky showings are light-hearted gatherings and far less intimidating that the full on S&M clubs or swinger's groups. Whether you go to see the film or the play, it is an opportunity to meet other ordinary individuals letting their hair down and gently pushing the boundaries of their inhibitions. For anybody that enjoys the costume role-play aspect of sexual fantasy, attending a Rocky Show is highly recommended.

For the purposes of bedroom fantasies let us imagine for a moment a culture or a planet in which women are the dominant sex. Perhaps we are many years into the future and radioactive mutation has caused female babies to grow into larger, stronger organisms than male babies. In five hundred years, this could make quite a difference. On the other hand, maybe women are as beautiful and desirable as they are now, but that, somehow, managed to achieve a dominant position. Perhaps they have learned a form of psychic mind-control techniques, or some genius woman inventor has invented a male 'pain collar' which can cause excruciating agony if they are not pleasing. If the collar is tampered with, the pain commences. Keys to these collars, or methods for removing them, are kept in secret, well-guarded places by well trained, heavily-armed women.

Along with the collars men would doubtless be put in confining garments and would be taught to smile, be pretty, and not challenge, but serve their mistresses. This particular male has come to the attention of the Imperious Queen. Her interest in the male slave, observed from her palanquin carried by eight muscular servants, is not platonic. It is sexual. He is as much a sex object to her as any woman could be to any man. He is ordered to her chambers where he becomes the helpless slave whose sole purpose is to please her. He soon discovers that just being 'loomed over' can induce a feeling of psychological helplessness.

Many women, have excellent reasons, at least from time to time, for resenting men and their dominance. This fantasy, then, allows a woman to ventilate these deep, and justified resentments. It allows her to be on top, to be dominant, to be the master. This can be thrilling to her. This is a scenario where men, not women, are kept in harems, controlled by robots, and female officers, who could destroy them at the slightest sign of disobedience.

Such fantasies are not uncommon to women. In a sense they are vengeance fantasies. It is very liberating for a woman to be permitted to enact them. If you love your partner presumably you will want her to have this cathartic, hostility-venting experience. She has many scores to settle with 'men,' and also, of course, with you personally. Much as you love one another, you will surely, from time to time, get on one another's nerves. The sweet, open discharge of hostility in the context of fantasy, concluding with mutual exquisite pleasure for both, is a fantastic experience. It is good for getting 'it' out of the system of both.

In all things, he must obey the will of his mistress. Whatever she wishes, he must do. If she wishes, he must kneel before her and put his head and lips to her feet. If she wishes, he must, commanded, crawl into her bed. Perhaps she would, first, desire him to wash her body, or her hair; perhaps he must comb her hair; perhaps he must bring her certain garments or adorn her, according to her directions; perhaps he is to read her Oriental love poetry; perhaps he is to prepare food for her and feed her; or fetch wine for her and, kneeling, serve it to her. Perhaps she will command him to wear certain garments; perhaps she will even order him to adorn himself with certain jewellery. Women, for example, are forced to be pleasing to men. Let a man feel what it is like to be forced to be pleasing to a woman. Let him learn to smile and to be submissive and ingratiating. It may give him a real insight into what it is to be a woman. It should make him more human.

A great advantage of this fantasy, incidentally, which should not be overlooked, is that the man responds to the woman's directions. She should, then, instruct him as to how to make love to her. She tells him where to touch her and how. This can be extremely valuable to the male in informing him as to what excites her. It can also be liberating to the female because, in the context of the fantasy, she must command him.

In standard sex she might be reticent to say what she wants. In a world of fantasy, she is much more likely to give him detailed and explicit directions. It allows her, in the fantasy, to communicate her wants and her needs. Later, of course, in other situations, he should remember what pleased her. Furthermore, she, as queen or ruler, will insist on her complete pleasure. For example, she may not permit the male, under her command, to penetrate her until she is, an hour or so later, on her final orgasm. When penetration does take place presumably she will kneel across his body, writhing, taking him. Let him lie on his back this time. Let him look up at the dominant partner, who uses him for her pleasure.

For an unexpected twist, the man can take the role of a female slave, and the woman of the male master. There are four logical relations which are worth exploring in this type of fantasy. Consider the role of the female slave first as the male wishes the role played, and, secondly, as the female feels it is ideally played. For example, the male might wish the female-slave role played as a girl who, cringing and overwhelmed, stunned, knows her master at the first sight of him, and the female, though ultimately wishing to be completely conquered, wishes it to be a real battle for him, wishing to act the role of a proud, independent girl who though entrapped helplessly in the institution of slavery nonetheless tries to retain a shred of dignity until at last it is forced from her and she yields, and totally, submitting to her master. There are no reasons, of course, why there can not be many varieties of female slave, depending on their backgrounds, etc.

Consider the role of the male master first as the male wishes the role played, and, secondly, as the female feels it is ideally played. For example, perhaps the male wishes to play it casually, insulting his wench by taking her for granted, and the female might wish it played much more dominantly, more cruelly, more ruthlessly, paying her more attention as a helpless object to be dominated. She might wish her master to be the sort of man who takes her by the hair and throws her to his feet, scornfully, at whose feet, in terror, she is forced to kneel, head down. Perhaps only such a man, who is ruthless and powerful, uncompromising, would be strong enough to dominate her. There are no reasons, of course, why there can not be many varieties of male master, depending on their backgrounds.

The four possibilities here then are that she directs him as female and herself as male, directing both roles; that he directs himself as female and she as male, directing both roles; that she directs him as female and he directs her as male; and that he directs himself as female and she directs herself as male. This sort of thing works out best, incidentally, when there is considerable discussion prior to any attempted performance. This fantasy, however, can deepen and enrich one's conception of both roles and can be a delight. This fantasy, incidentally, can have a bonus for the woman. Most women tend to feel hostility not only once in a while for men, but also, interestingly, toward other women. This might also be enjoyable for her to do to some female she dislikes, her husband acting that role, she acting the role of a rough, ruthless man who makes her respond to him, and 'puts her in her place.'

30. ROMAN ORGIES

The Romans were notorious for their enormous sexual appetites. Their culture was very different to our own and sex played a large part in their liberal and uninhibited lifestyles. Later Christians may have exaggerated their degree of depravity, and there is a good chance that the most immoral, disgusting behaviours were rumours made up by political enemies or gossiping plebs, but a little romantic role play as Caesar and Cleopatra can still be very exciting.

There are many iconic roles with which to experiment but a good place to start is a small, private Roman banquet. This can give you a taste of the licentious atmosphere of their Bacchanalian feasts and help you decide if this is an era in which you would like to explore more of your sexual fantasies. Imported from Greece, the Bacchanalia were 'fertility festivals' that really took hold in modern South Italy. Writing about these 'festivals' in the Augustan era, the historian Livy breathlessly described scenes of unimaginable debauchery. These 'festivals' were alleged to be a place where people met, danced themselves into ecstasy, then fell into frantic copulation with no regard for who or what they might be screwing. This is not just Livy going on a fantasy-trip, either. By all accounts, the authorities were so troubled by the practice that they outlawed them, with punishments of severe torture imposed on anyone who continued to practice. Remember this is Rome, at the height of its decadence – so anything they want to ban as 'immoral' has got to be pretty extreme. Yet, for all the threat of torture lingered over its followers, the cult of Bacchus survived for centuries – along with its pervy, orgiastic rites.

To recreate the Roman era in you own home, treat yourselves to a selection of exotic delicacies along with a few delicious drinks and arrange them on a low table surrounded by cushions. I like to choose a range of tastes as well as foods with interesting textures. The Romans were not big on knives and forks so everything will be finger foods at this meal. The radish especially had very sexual overtones during the Roman period and vegetables were often used as sex toys. For some strange reason, lettuce was considered to be a Viagra of the time. Select sweets as well as savouries and choose your accompanying drinks carefully too. A novel liqueur makes a fine substitute for imported spiced wines, collected from the far flung corners of Empire. Add a few contemporary standards such as olives and grapes for a touch of authenticity. Try to avoid overly processed food that will take away from the realism.

The master or mistress of the house should be wearing a toga for the sake of modesty. Most of us have been to toga parties and know how easy it is to convert a simply sheet into a senatorial Roman robe. Accessorise with a few large costume jewellery rings and some sandals for added effect. The slave will have a simple and brief tunic, tied at the waist and fastened on the left shoulder by a golden clasp. Even the Romans were not above equipping their house slaves with a collar and chain. Well-endowed slaves would be forced to keep the prowess on show at all times; and images of the fertility God Priapus weighing his own gigantic member would appear over the entrance of houses as a form of good luck. They certainly did not have the advantages of electricity so try to find an oil lamp or if that is not available, eat by candlelight. Download some lyre music that can be played in the background while to eat. I would recommend the 'Ancient Romans' by Sun Araw and 'Lyre 'n' Rhapsody' by Awakening the Muse.

Imagine that you are the Master of the house, on a visit to your villa after a long stationing at the front. For many seasons you and your legionnaires have been fending off the attacks of the barbarian hordes. At last you are back in Rome, ready to enjoy the spoils of war. You are fascinated with this new slave that is now serving you. Did you capture her yourself on your most recent campaign, binding and leashing her in the streets of a burning city? Was she perhaps the daughter of a conquered chieftain, chained with her other women in their burning palisade, before being led to the locked slave carts, or being tied by the neck to your stirrup? Maybe you purchased her at the market? Was it your bid that took her naked off the block? Was she a bargain or did you pay much more than you originally intended, and you now feel hostile toward her? Doubtless you are determined to get more than your money's worth. Or did your servants bring her home, hoping that she might please you? Is this the first time you have seen her, as she brings food to you? Did an old friend from the Senate give her to you as a welcome home gift? Now, again, look at her, again closely, very closely, as she serves you. Command her; she is yours to do with as you please. When, during the banquet, you want her, you tear away her her flimsy garment. You can command her to dance for you. You can yank her roughly by the chain and pull her down onto the cushions beside you to see if she will yield well to her new master. Possibly you will need to teach her the ways of her new household. This might include punishment for poor performance or lack of etiquette. If she is a barbarian wench from a vanquished kingdom then maybe she will need extended training to meet your expectations. If she is impertinent then maybe she will need the lash to make her more compliant. Most slaves were war captives, sold as property to the Roman citizenry. A slave of Rome had absolutely no rights and was utterly at the mercy of his/her master (a situation known as 'dominica potestas'), who could use them for sexual gratification and have them flogged or killed as they pleased.

Many Romans kept beautiful slaves as deliciae or delicati ('sweets, dainties') a term that is often applied to slaves used specifically for sexual gratification and companionship. A Roman could exploit his own slaves for sex, but was not entitled to compel any enslaved person he chose to have sex, since the owner had the right to control his own property. In the pursuit of sex with a slave who belonged to someone else, persuasion or threats might be employed. A charge of rape could not be brought against a free man who forced a slave to have sex, since a slave lacked the legal standing that protected a citizen's body, but the owner could prosecute the rapist under the Lex Aquilia, a law pertaining to property damage.

One notorious banquet was arranged for the Consul Metellus Scipio by Gemellus, the tribunicial errand boy. He was originally a free man by birth, but compelled in business to play the servant's role. Society gave a collective blush when he established a whorehouse in his own home, and pimped out Mucia and Flavia, each of them notable for her father and husband, along with the aristocratic boy Saturninus. The People's Tribunes enjoyed countless young bodies in shameless submission, performing outrageous games of drunken sex.

Prostitution was both legal and tolerated, and common place. Whenever the Emperor Nero sailed down the Tiber to Ostia, for example, booths were set up at intervals along the banks and shores, completely fitted out for commercial debauchery. The arches under the circus of the Colosseum were known as fornices (arcade dens) were often used as brothels where the prostitutes were slaves or freed-women. This gave us the Latin root of the word fornication. In general, brothels were rough places and strictly for the lower classes. Roman elites preferred to bring the brothel to them and had whole wings of their villas dedicated to carnal pleasures. Bath house were not the dens of iniquity that we might suppose. Imperial Rome established edicts against the mingling of genders in public baths. This meant that straight men and women at least had to find alternative locations for their trysts. Gardens and alleys were popular.

The existence of sex clubs may provide background for Late Republican political smears about public figures whose party guests included many prostitutes and courtesans. None was more famous than the Imperial whorehouse Caligula established on the Palatine, where he prostituted married women and freeborn youths. Group sex appears in literary sources, graffiti, and art. Suetonius says that the emperor Tiberius enjoyed watching group sex, and described 'chains' arranged of girls and boys: In his retreat at Capri, he put together a bedroom that was the theatre of his secret debauches. There he assembled from all over companies of male and female prostitutes, and inventors of monstrous couplings (which he called spintriae), so that, intertwining themselves and forming a triple chain (triplici serie connexi), they mutually prostituted themselves in front of him to fire up his flagging desires.

Of course you need not indulge in full scale Roman orgies to taste the pleasures of the ancient world. Gladiators were the rock stars of their day and attracted more than fair share of groupies. The female mistresses of gladiators were called 'ludia' and were regarded with the same mixture of fascination and contempt given in the 1920s to gangsters' molls. It was not uncommon for a wayward noblewoman to elope with a famous gladiator, and this was a scandalous event that delighted the public. After a full day of slaughtering wild beasts and massacring Christians, every gladiator needs a long relaxing massage or perhaps a good soak in the tub to wash away all that blood. Why not try a little olive oil for an after-circus rub-down.

31. ROUGH SEX

Not all women have the same type of ravishment fantasies. While some may prefer the more violent, spontaneous type of scenarios, others prefer something that is a little more akin to a slightly forceful seduction and is a little more planned. Some adore the feeling of being pushed up against a wall. Not necessarily to have sex, just shoved up against a wall and made out with. Out of passion, not anger. It is so sexy to be held against a wall by someone who you do not think will hurt you. Slam her against the wall, make out with her, throw her on the bed and have your wicked way.

While some women do fantasise about being brutally raped, other just want their boyfriend to go from his normal sweet, loving self to a total masculine, lustful beast that just cannot take his hands off of her. Force her into your bedroom by walking forward without stopping, physically forcing her to take steps backward without touching her. Man-handle her in a hot and sexy way, never taking your eyes off her, fully focused on both your and her sexual fulfillment. There is no rush, just make it very intense. Take the lead, sweep her away completely with your passion when you do have your way with her she will completely surrender to you. There is something in a woman that wants to surrender itself to a strong, desirable male. In a sense, sexually, a woman does frequently want to be dominated. Women who fantasize the victim role imagine being forced into sexual situations against their will. They are sexually excited at the idea of being completely controlled and dominated.

The notion of being taken by force is another common fantasy. Sometimes blended with the "stranger" theme or a desire for domination. Force can be as benign as raising her arms over her head and making love against a wall – passionately, where the operative term is passion, not violence. The man's ardour is fuelled by the woman's response, and her response, by his primal need to have her. Rape fantasies do not always involve men. One woman I knew described a situation which took place near the ocean. She explained the ocean is a huge powerful force, and she was afraid of it. It would overwhelm her. It threatened her and so the only way for her to deal with it was to open her legs.

The following extract is a ravishment fantasy from the Nancy Friday book series.

He forcibly pushes me against the wall and pins my arms above my head with one hand while the other hand makes its way under my skirt and fondles my vagina. The man rips off my clothes, forces open my legs, penetrates me, and concurrently smears my lipstick all over my face with his forceful kiss.

This is why a woman will jump for joy when you can pull this one through for her. The key is not to be much concerned for her pleasure. Women get off when a man desires her so much that he just uses her body as something to fuck and give himself pleasure. When you are turned on and going crazy with lust, she is turned on and going crazy too. Your state will automatically lead her state. To do a ravishment be extremely commanding. Do not ask her what she likes. Do not ask her what she wants. Just tell her what you want and do not use a lot of words to do it. Actions speak louder than words. Fuck her hard like you just got out of prison and she is the first girl you have seen. Ravish her from the depths of your core. Lead strongly and command her in the direction you want to go. It is key for you to get into the right state of mind. For a woman to feel ravished, you need to be in the mental state of a ravisher. Imagine this woman is your illicit mistress and you are going to devour her body. Imagine you have never been attracted to someone so physically and you will fuck her from the very depths of your being with intense and uninhibited lust. Grab her by the waist and start making out with her. Lift her arms over her head. Push her up against the well. Lift her up and throw her on a piece of furniture. It does not have to happen in the bedroom. Too many couples only have sex in the bedroom. If you truly wanted to ravish your woman, you would not wait for the bedroom. You would take her right there in the kitchen or anywhere else. Lick her face. Kiss her all over and hungrily grope her tits. Start off like you are holding back your desire, like there is a flood gate about to explode. Tell her, you want to fuck you so bad that you can barely contain yourself. Rip off her clothes and handle her body roughly with your hands. Treat her like a piece of meat, like her sole purpose is to get you off. Do not be afraid to get a little messy and leave sweat and drool all over her body. Start talking sexy to her in every manner as you devour her body. If you catch her off guard, she may not be in the mood, but if your passion is strong enough, it can put her into the mood. As the ravisher it is your job to be relentless, to not give up, to punch through the wall until the woman submits and surrenders to your passions.

Rough sex is a sexual release where you can show off your brute strength and your lust at the same time. Rough sex is not something most people talk about easily, but yet, it is something all of us could enjoy if done the right way. If you are not someone who is into rough sex, bringing all that aggression into something as romantic as lovemaking could sound alarming, but that will all change once you understand the little nuances of passionate rough sex here. Firstly, rough sex is best enjoyed with a partner you trust. Both of you know each other's limitations and capabilities, and it is easy to know where to draw the line. If you claw your lover's back with your nails, the rage they experience will subconsciously force them to reciprocate your rough moves with their own, which can lead to a heightened sexual experience for both of you. When you are genuinely having rough sex, the urge to enhance the sexual sensation is so overwhelming that even penetration cannot satisfy you. You want to do more. It hurts but you like it, and that is what makes the whole thing so passionate. There is something about a man's physical strength and animal-like aggression that can awe a girl.

When you have rough sex with your girl, it shows off your confidence and your manly, wild side which can turn her on and rekindle the raw sexual desire in her. But how rough would she like it? Start slow by kissing more aggressively and using your teeth, but as you get more into the act, apply more pressure on your partner, either by using your hands or your pelvis. Run your hands through your lover's hair and grip it firmly with your fingers while whispering something dirty or biting your lover's neck. Nibble and bite. Using teeth is always a great way to bring out the animal in you when you are in bed. Bite hard, but not hard enough to draw blood. Focus on erogenous zones like the neck, the breasts, belly, inner thighs and around the elbows and ankles. And when you feel comfortable enough, run your nails against your partner's back, deeper with each confident thrust of your pelvis. And somewhere along the way, you will start to feel the wild passion engulf you. And before you know it, you will be all roughed up and ready for a wild, rough time in bed. Pain and pleasure release endorphins, a morphine-like chemical created in the body. If you learn to mix pain with sexual pleasure while having rough sex, you would be able to experience more of the feel good sensation instantly. Not all of us are sexual screamers. But when you get roughed up and shed your vocal inhibitions enough to scream and yell, you will feel more relaxed and carefree, which will make you wilder. Scratch and claw with your fingernails. Running a painful line with your fingernails against the soft skin of your lover's back will send a sexy rush that can cause a lot of pain too. But when you are on a sexual high, all that pain will turn to sexual adrenalin. Pull each other's hair. Grab a handful of your lover's hair just above the scalp at the back of the head, and tug at it. You will not lose your grip and yet, the pain will feel more pleasurable than when you hold your lover by the lower ends of their hair. Pound each other like there is no tomorrow, and the aggressive to-and-fro movements will turn both of you on, just as long as both of you can hold on long enough. But remember, you are dealing with fragile body parts here, so do not get carried away and push too deep or too hard. Slap each other across the face or the chest, or if you are standing behind your partner who is on all fours, slap their back or their butt. The searing pain will bring out the animal in your lover. Ever heard the lines, "Say my name!" or "Call me a bitch!"? Well, many lovers love getting called trashy names and hearing dirty abuse. If your lover enjoys being called a whore, go ahead and indulge them.

Being aware of some of the things that can go wrong will help you to avoid painful, uncomfortable outcomes. If a girl sits down heavily or the guy aggressively penetrates deep, broken penis is definitely possible. Penetrating too deep in a hurried motion can damage a girl's cervix which can lead to bleeding or bruising. It is difficult to control ejaculation and orgasms while having rough sex. Your protection can get damaged while doing the rough nasty. Tears in the vaginal walls are due to aggressive rough sex. Even worse, tearing of the skin on the male can be life threatening due to severe blood loss, so be careful about going to hard without any lubrication. If you notice any painful swellings or bleeding after rough sex, consult your doctor, especially if the symptoms last for more than a couple of days. Of course none of this should be a problem if you slammed her up against the wall and followed all of the other advice above.

32. SACRED SEXUALITY

Descriptions of the ancient world are filled with stories of fertility temples and beautiful priestesses. Some of the first societies to emerge along the banks of the Tigris and Euphrates rivers featured many such 'houses of heaven.' According to the 5th-century BC historian Herodotus, the rites performed at these temples included sacred sex, or what scholars later called sacred prostitution. He described a Babylonian custom in which every woman of the land would sit in the temple of Aphrodite and offer herself to the faithful. These ranged from the richest and most powerful royals who arrived at the temple in covered carriages drawn by teams, accompanied by a great retinue of attendants. Ordinary women were seated in the sacred plot of Aphrodite, with crowns of cord on their heads; there was a great multitude of women coming and going; passages filled by the men who passed to make their choice. They cast coins into her lap and recited the phrase "I invite you in the name of Mylitta" (the Assyrian name for Aphrodite). It did not matter what sum the money was; the woman would never refuse, for that would be a sin, the money being sacred. Following their union, and having discharged her sacred duty to the goddess, she was free to return to her home. The women that were fair and tall were soon free to depart, but the uncomely may have had a long wait; some of them might have remained for years.

The Ancient Kings of Sumer established their legitimacy by taking part in a ritual sexual act in the temple of the fertility goddess Ishtar every year on the tenth day of the New Year festival Akitu. This 'sacred marriage' ritual was between the King and the High Priestess of Inanna, the Sumerian goddess of sexual love, fertility, and warfare. The greatest temple dedicated to Inanna was situated in Uruk. The Akkadian counterpart of Inanna was Ishtar, and the Canaanite equivalent was Astarte, whom the Greeks accepted under the name of Aphrodite. The Roman equivalent was Venus.

185

The Hebrew Bible refers to qedesha or consecrated holy prostitute. These were common among the Canaanites. In the Book of Ezekiel, Oholah and Oholibah appear as the allegorical brides of God who represent Samaria and Jerusalem. They became prostitutes in Egypt, engaging in prostitution from their youth.

According to the contemporary Christian writer Eusebius, the Phoenician cities of Aphaca and Heliopolis (Baalbek) continued to practice temple prostitution until the emperor Constantine closed down the rite in the 4th century AD. In Ancient Greece, sacred prostitution was known in the city of Corinth where the temple of Aphrodite employed a significant number of female servants, hetairai, during classical antiquity.

In some parts of ancient India, women competed to win the title of Nagarvadhu or 'Bride of the City.' The most beautiful woman was chosen and was respected as a goddess. She served as a courtesan, and the price for a single night's dance was very high, within reach only for the king, the princes and the lords.

For some variety on this theme, the Mayans maintained several phallic religious cults involving homosexual temple prostitution. Aztec religious leaders were heterosexually celibate and engaged in homosexuality with one another as a religious practice, temple idols were often depicted engaging in homosexuality, and the god Xochipili was both the patron of homosexuals and homosexual prostitutes. The Inca sometimes dedicated young boys as temple prostitutes. The boys were dressed in girls clothing, and chiefs and headmen would have ritual homosexual intercourse with them during religious ceremonies and on holidays. This could make for an interesting role reversal fantasy with a chance to try out some forays into pegging. In addition, Xochiquetzal was worshipped as goddess of sexual power, patroness of prostitutes and artisans involved in the manufacture of luxury items.

All of these stories offer plenty of inspiration for some exciting and exotic costumed role-play. If you are in Europe where barrow mounds and monolithic standing stones are more common than Aztec pyramids and Greek temples then remember that in Irish Mythology

Clíodhna was an sometimes depicted as Queen of the Banshees but also as the goddess of love. Stonehenge probably has to many tourists most of the time but if you are there at the solstice, I would imagine that such open fertility rites might even be actively encouraged for those with a strong streak of exhibitionism.

For something that is well beyond the imagination of normal folks, I highly recommend the 'The Planet of Adventure' by that master of fantasy, Jack Vance. The climax of the fifth chapter takes place in the Fasm Seminary of the Female Mystery, a setting so bizarre that it makes the perversions of the Hellfire Club and the excesses of the Bullingdon Boys appear extremely tame in comparison.

33. Upstairs, Downstairs, in my Lady's Chamber

While few people employ servants in their own homes anymore, staying in a hotel is often a great opportunity to indulge in a few butler or maid fantasies. Many a traveller has fantasised about a surprise visit from a a sexy French maid and being offered considerably more than the regular housekeeping services. This can easily be bought to life, especially if your partner has one of those wonderful maid outfits. Have her pose as the hotel maid and walk in on you just as you are emerging from the shower. If she has a few props to add some realism then all the better. A spray bottle and an armful of extra towels should do the trick and a feather duster can be put to all kinds of imaginative uses. Asian parents tend to use these as the default home implement to beat their children and so these can get Chinese girls especially extremely aroused.

The hotel patron will be busy in the shower when the maid comes in to clean. He will not even notice at first that she has stopped working and started admiring his wet, naked body. But somehow, she gives herself away. Perhaps she peeks around the shower curtain and is spotted. Perhaps she gives him a well-deserved compliment: and he hears it. Perhaps their hands touch as he reaches for a towel just as she is restocking the rack. However the connection is made, the scene ends with her removing her uniform and joining him for some splashy fun. The maid might walk in to find her hotel bed occupied by a naked and horny guest. Maybe some hotel porn is playing on the television. If you are both feeling extra-bold, he could even be in the middle of stroking off when she busts in. She is blushing and apologetic, of course, to have interrupted at such a delicate moment. But as it turns out, her company is not at all unwelcome. Invite her to sit down and watch the porno or the jack-off show. Maybe she will ask if she can touch it. Maybe she will need a little more reassurance first, like a back rub and a shower of compliments. Promise not to tell her boss. You two can take it from here. Especially good for voyeurs and exhibitionists.

Perhaps while the maid is cleaning, she finds some sex toys in the night stand drawer. These could consist of a small vibrator or a cock ring, or maybe a blindfold and some bondage ties: it is up to you and what kind of sex play you are planning for later. Now it is the hotel guest's turn to be a bit embarrassed and apologetic. At least until she asks for a demonstration. Who would turn down an opportunity like this? This role play gives her a chance to act as the seducer instead of the seduced, plus it provides both of you lots of opportunities to experiment with your toys.

In an older hotel, with some suitably vintage clothing it is quite easy to get down and dirty, Downton Abbey style with a helpless maid type fantasy. For him a smoking jacket, a monocle and a pipe would suffice all the way up to spats and tails if you fancy your self as a bit of a Bertie Wooster. If she has a French maid outfit, then the pair of you could always going to a midnight showing of the Rocky Horror Show as an encore.

For the moment, the maid discovers her employer not to be the kind of English gentleman that she was originally led to believe. Many unfortunate girls in past generations, have found themselves in this sort of predicament. Jobs were very scarce, and a good position in a rich household was very desirable. A young woman who wishes to retain her employment, might discover it would be well for her to sleep with the master. There were plenty of girls willing to take her place.

In many fantasies, it is helpful to engage in activities that help one to get in the mood for the fantasy, and, indeed, might even be considered as an introductory portion of the fantasy. If she is not a housewife, but has a maid, she can dismiss the real maid early and perform some of her tasks herself, to get into the mood. She can meet the partner at the door, take his hat, address him as "Sir," and so on. All day long, we may suppose, she has, in fear, anticipated that he will indicate his desire to her that she serve him sexually. What will she do? She does not know. She is in agony. He is, of course, handsome and strong, and sexually attractive to her. After supper, she will see what happens. But, after supper, he asks her nothing. He merely begins to remove her clothing. "Sir!" she exclaims. But, overwhelmed, stunned, helpless before his boldness, obedient, she is lifted naked and carried to the bed.

The benefit of a set of tails over a smoking jacket is that the male can then play the role of handsome butler. I do not mean that hideously hairless oddball from the Rocky Horror Freakshow but a diligent and meticulous male servant of the highest order. After turning down the covers, he might be required to turn on the more than just the electric blanket.

34. SEX – ONE MILLION YEARS BC

A cave girl is caught and dragged to the cave of her captor, an aggressive neolithic caveman. She is dragged inside and there is no escape. In the back of the cave, in the dim, flickering light, on the furs, she is on her hands and knees, or she crouches against the back wall, in terror, a trapped female. Her captor squats in the entrance of the cave, regarding her. After a time, he approaches her. He tears her garment from her. On the furs, in the light of the small fire, amidst the wild shadows, as she struggles, he brutalises her. When he is finished with her, she does not desire to leave him. She puts her head against his body. She wishes to be permitted to remain, to be his mate.

This standard troglodyte fantasy, is so common and familiar that it has been delightfully satirized for many years. We are all familiar with the cartoon of the cave man whacking his beauty over the head with a club and dragging her to his cave. Of course, if you intend to enact this fantasy, leave out the clubbing part. On the other hand, hair yanking or physical brutality and dragging her about, can all be very exciting. Many women find a little pain, psychic or physical, sexually stimulating. Their favourite fantasy is not the rape fantasy for nothing. The familiarity of the fantasy speaks its general power; if it were not as powerful and widespread as it is, it would not be so familiar.

For this fantasy to be maximally effective, it is important for both partners to psychically impart themselves into the entire situation. They must think and feel the whole situation. There is no civilization. There is no rule of law, only lust and force. Moralities, scruples, restraints, do not exist. There are no polite marriage ceremonies. Mating is by capture. No social artifices, no glosses, no contracts, no meaningless rituals. The victim's plight is that she will be sexually subjugated by her captor. The primitive realities of the time are that if he wants her, he will have her. This is a raw fantasy, and a very exciting one for those who dare to enact it. Perhaps the female is bound hand and foot with rawhide thongs and carried to the cave? (Rawhide boot-straps make superb binding thongs for women.) She is at the mercy of the man who has captured her. She is helpless. He can do what he wants with her. There is very little developed language. It is very important, to understand the rawness and primitiveness of the world in which these individuals find themselves. Candlelight can add a great deal to this scenario as can a few fake furs from the thrift store. It is difficult to pull off the illusion of being a true cave dweller in Levis and a plaid shirt. A roughly hewn stick can take the place of a stone club. My own predilection is to feed the bound female, giving her a sense of comfort before I turn back into a lustful brute, seemingly incapable of compassion. It certainly heightens the experience. The fact that this may according to anthropologists be an inaccurate depiction of the early palaeolithic era is unimportant.

There has been some speculation that the wedding ring is symbolically reminiscent of the bonds in which the captive female is placed. There is also a suggestion that the act of a husband carrying his wife over the threshold of his home is also a throwback to this kind of capture. The act seems symbolically reminiscent of capture and carrying the female into one's stronghold, whether it is a cave or a castle, or 27B King's Close. Ironically it seems that the reality is that primate societies were much more likely to be matriarchal than a leadership of strong, dominant males. Books such as the Chalice and the Blade by Rianne Eisler seriously challenge our widespread beliefs about male dominated hierarchies of the past. Even so, there are still primitive tribes today, that regard females as suitable objects of predation. Recorded history (written mainly by male predators) is replete with tales of capture, rape and enslavement of human females. It is a scenario that has been force fed to us by story tellers for many years now and that is one reason why it makes for such an excellent sexual fantasy.

An interesting variant is to imagine the woman as a highly educated, brilliant, modern woman, perhaps a scientist doing field work in a very remote part of the jungle. This is reminiscent of the classic Tarzan fantasy. She finds herself, a modern woman, hunted, caught and mated. She is introduced into the savage life of the tribe, forced to do the servile, repetitive work allotted to the cave females. She must, with other women, and children, and dogs, remain at the camp, while the men hunt, and make war. When her cave-man master returns, he uses her sexually, with gusto. Perhaps the camp is raided, and she, with others, are carried off to be the slaves of other cave men. Doubtless she is beaten and bound, and forced to be pleasing. Perhaps then she is rescued.

Of course, the female can always reverse the roles here and become the Amazon warrior princess, the Barsoomian queen. She has trapped a prize specimen of the male species and she will now bend him to her will. If he is proud and strong, he will need to be broken, subjugated and humiliated until he realises that he is now her plaything, with whom she can do whatever she wishes.

35. Spies, Counterspies and Assassins

The Ian Fleming fantasy world of spies has for a long time been extremely glamorous and highly sexually charged. Most of us have grown up with these romps, shown on TV, as they were on every bank holiday celebration. There has since become something innately sexual about a man in a tuxedo and a femme-fatale female counter-spy.

A basic interrogation scene might start out with the spymaster 'capturing' and forcibly restraining a counter intelligence agent, perhaps by stripping them and tying them to a chair or to the bed. If the captive is tied to a chair, this can be a very simple attachment, just tied wrists behind the chair back is sufficient. If you wish to tie ankles to chair legs for added effect then by all means feel free. This works especially well if the captive is wearing a seductive or even skimpy outfit. Imagine the captive's shock as a stiletto flick-knife snaps open just in front of her eyes and then begins cutting away the buttons from a tight blouse, one by excruciating one. In many locations a good flick knife is hard to find and so it is perfectly acceptable to make do with a pair of scissors. The trick here is to make sure that they are completely unfamiliar to the captive. Nothing kills a fantasy as quickly as the appearance of a pair of easily recognised kitchen scissors. Far more convincing is a menacing pair of long-nosed surgical scissors, purchased especially for the purpose. These are even more effective if you are willing to cut the captive out of their clothes rather than simply remove them in the normal fashion. Once a cut has been made at the edge of piece of fabric, it will tear much more easily. This means that once buttons have slowly and teasingly been removed, the remaining garments can be energetically ripped away. This kind of contrast works very well to make the fantasy so much more real and therefore sexually exciting. Once the clothing has been removed, you can repeatedly tease the captive to the brink of orgasm, stopping a few times before driving them over the edge.

The extraction of classified information can take as long as the captive agent wishes to hold out. An effective strategy in this case is for the spy to have hidden away an envelope marked Top Secret somewhere in the very near vicinity. It need only contain a photo but it could also hold a diary or even a code book of secret information for added extra realism. I like to use a page of complex mathematical formulae that I have copied from the internet. This is usually meaningless to both participants but suggests that captive is a highly intelligent operative, moving in the very highest echelons of industrial espionage. This way the spy can decide for themselves how long they wish to submit out, depending on how much they are enjoying the processing. They can wriggle and writhe for as long as they are enjoying the experience.

The spy master then begins 'torturing' the captured agent to obtain the information. This 'torture' can combine many aspects: clothes pegs, spanking, paddling, mock 'rape,' and so on. If the agent refuses turn over the information, the interrogator can keep escalating the interrogation, gradually moving to more and more intense activity, until the operative cracks and reveals all.

The key to an effective session of this nature is to keep it all very Hollywood. Think back to the famous laser table scene in the classic 007 movie, Goldfinger. Bond is uncomfortably spread eagled and asks his captor,

"Do you expect me to talk?"

"No Mr. Bond," the villain responds "I expect you to die!"

In our scenario, this could be changed to "No my dear, I expect you you to squirt."

Focus on the imminent threat of pain and discomfort while refraining from from any actual physical mistreatment. The psychological aspect is far more stimulating. Running the tips of scissors across naked flesh is extremely arousing. For added effect blindfold the captive and then explore then tenderest parts of the body with a feather or a finely tipped brush. Of course, if the captive has a liking for pain then the processing procedures can be altered to meet their requirements. Bear in mind though that not everybody has masochist tendencies and that on most people the suggestion of torture is far more exciting that any real infliction. As in all fantasies, care must be taken not to injure or frighten a partner. There is nothing desirable about pain, fear and misery.

As always, think about appealing to as many of the senses as possible in this scenario. Lighting is relatively easy to alter. Most people will have some kind of lamp that can be used as an interrogation spot light. If not then candlelight always harks back to a harsh dungeon environment. This also adds a sense of smell to add further effect to the proceedings.

This scenario is so well ingrained into our consciousness, that it is relatively easy to select costumes that will enhance the experience. Regardless of what goes on the real world, fantasy special agents are glamorous and chic. For women this can mean any kind of party dress. For men a tuxedo is the first choice, but a turtle neck sweater and a blazer will make a perfectly acceptable substitute. For props think about a pipe, a cigarette case or maybe even an eye-patch. For ladies a cigarette holder is perfect. Remember to refer to each other with suitably spy like stage names. For women this is usually Daphne or Penelope. For men, a hereditary title is often very effective. Of course you could always utilise that tension that has been built up over the last fifty years between a simple 'James' and 'Money-penny'

Thanks to 007, everybody knows what a male MI5 operative should like like. For a female role model it is necessary to look a little further back in time. The femme-fatale, Mata Hari, occupies a particularly romantic spot in the annals of international espionage. Before the First World War, she made her living as a dancer. Her sultry features and almond eyes supported her claims of Oriental ancestry. Mata Hari claimed to have grown up on Java, where she had learned the sacred temple dances and became a priestess in the cult of Siva. The beautiful dancer acquired many wealthy lovers, some of whom held high ranks in the military. She did in fact hail from Holland. Her real name was Margaret Gertrud Macleod, and the only time that she had spent in Java was as the battered wife of a drunken Army captain, who served as a colonial administrator. Upon her return to Europe, she reinvented herself and began to turn her power over men to good advantage. She went to and fro as a spy and counter-spy for almost every major power in Europe. After a slew of lovers, adventures and and intrigues, she was eventually sentenced to death by the French. Facing a firing squad of twelve riflemen, she refused a blindfold and was executed on October 15, 1917. Tales remain to this day that it was a mock execution and that she feigned death only to be resccued by one of her many high-ranking lovers.

Once the captive has been thoroughly interrogated, broken both mentally and physically, then they should be drugged and crated. While I do not recommend the actual use of a syringe for any kind of injection, they do make an exciting prop with which to threaten the victim. Syringes can easily become contaminated, and they are also extremely dangerous with respect to the introduction of air into the system. Even so, as a theatrical device they evoke an instant and instinctive response in the same way that snakes or spiders do. If the captive is blindfolded then the effect can be even more powerful. Let them see the syringe before there eyes are covered. Then describe how you are going to give them an injection but instead of using a syringe, swab the area of bare flesh and then prick it with a pin. This is usually more than enough to convince a blindfolded captive that they have actually been injected. The use of a blindfold allows for the introduction of many elaborate illusions. A rubber snake can become terrifyingly real if used carefully on a captive whose vision has been restricted, especially if you can make convincing sound effects to go with it. My favourite version of this is the electric mosquito killer as a punishment tool. See Appendix 2 for more details.

When drugging and crating a captive, no actual drug is necessary. Imagination is more than sufficient. Similarly, presumably no 'crating' actually occurs, though a large cardboard box, if one is available, can always be a lot of fun. Make sure that there are sufficient air-holes of course. Think back to the hours of fun that had as a youngster when making dens and castles from ordinary cardboard boxes. That kind of childish pleasure can easily be recreated in the bedroom with much more adult themes.

She is shipped off to an alpine stronghold or perhaps the villain's lair is deep within the Tibetan Himalayas. Her skimpy garments do not permit her escape across the bleak, snow-swept mountains. The mountains themselves are the walls of her prison. Imagine the humiliation of a beautiful, intelligent female espionage agent, captured, forced to perform as a maid and sex slave. For example, she might be forced to make the bed, perfectly, and then to remove her clothing and get in it. Afterwards, perhaps, she may be expected to again change the linen. Perhaps the guest in the room commands her to dust or vacuum the room naked, perhaps while hobbled.

A variant on this type of fantasy is that in which the lovely spy, thinking she is to obtain secret information, accompanies a male agent to this 'mysterious hotel' in the mountains, thinking to buy secrets with the pleasures of her body. The pleasures of her body, as she learns, are then completely at the disposal of her enemies. She has been lured into a trap. She has been outwitted and tricked. You can continue this type of fantasy indefinitely, of course. Perhaps, somehow, the girl does manage to escape. Perhaps she is pursued. Perhaps, in a foreign capital, months later, she is again apprehended, kidnapped, and returned to her duties.

Yet another variant is a much more militarised version of the same theme. Imagine for example a resistance fighter has been captured by the local garrison - tied to a chair and interrogated as to the location of the secret base. Alternatively a soldier has been caught by the local guerrillas, who are known for their ruthless treatment of the Occupation forces. These offer two simple costume choices. This can be either a 'uniform' of dark green work pants, T-shirt and combat boots while she wears a partisenne costume of satin skirt, striped T-shirt, beret, and heels. Or he wears the beret and stripes as the Partisan while she wears a military-looking skirted suit with brass decorations and boots. Pick a war, pick a side, have fun with it. The interrogation might not always go as planned. Sometimes the captive may manage to seduce the guard and escape.

36. Supernatural Encounters

Spectrophiliac is the medical term that is used to describe spectre fetishists. In recent times these are the folks that have seen the movie Ghost too many times and now think of Patrick Swayze as a sexy, supernatural porn star. The reality is that this fetish has gone on throughout the centuries. While history is dotted with many stories of being raped by malevolent poltergeists, there are just as many romantic tales involving sensitive spirit lovers. While spectrophiles can always use their imagination for self satisfaction, most people who have this fetish really do believe they have had a sexual encounter with a ghost in the past. Many people who experience this phenomenon claim the ghost follows them throughout the rest of their lives.

For inspiration, there is a whole sub-genre of 'Invisible Man' porn in Japan. There again, there seems to be a sub-genre in Japan for just about every conceivable sexual kink. Perhaps an easier way to realise the ghost fantasy is simply to find some appropriately vintage costumes. This can range from simple sheets with eye holes cut out all the way to full Tudor courtier ensembles. I have attended a few cosplay conventions wearing the all black outfit and mask made famous by the Scream movies and the costume has proved to be extremely popular, as well as being instantly recognisable.

If you want to try recreating a ghostly sex scene. Here are a few tips. Atmosphere is all important. Candlelight is essential. Whisper your lover's name, so that it is barely audible. Run a trail of slender fingers down her spine and see if you can make her shiver. Use your breath to blow gently on the delicate areas of her body. Start with the backs of her arms and maybe her ankles. Try to create the feeling of ghostly fingers. All of this is much more effective if your partner is blindfolded the whole time. If she wants to keep her eyes open, there are plenty of ghost masks in the Halloween costume shops but in my experience a completely faceless mask is much more effective. Try one of those spandex masks that blanks out all the facial features. These can look very impressive in flickering candlelight. One very effective method is to straddle her chest so that she feels paralysed with a complete loss of control. Be careful not to suffocate here, but at least try to stifle her breathing.

In his book The Terror that Comes in the Night, folklorist David J. Hufford estimates that about 15 percent of people experience being assaulted in their sleep by an unknown entity at some point in their lives, often with a sexual element. In a 2012 radio interview with Ryan Seacrest, pop star Kesha talked about the inspiration for her song Supernatural, which involved 'Having sexy time with a ghost.' Lucy Liu and the late Anna Nicole Smith have also talked about having sex with spirit beings. St Teresa of Avila, who had more than her share of weird episodes, reportedly described a spirit encounters like this but sometimes it seems less naughty when it involves the Holy Ghost. Actually this was a large part of early Pagan religions. The practice was encouraged to create an earthly link between mortals and the gods, in order to guarantee fertile crops or good fortune. If you would like to learn more, paranormal researcher, Brad Steiger published a book of modern ghost sex stories called Sex and the Supernatural in 1968. More recently in 2012, the Travel Channel aired a documentary called Ghostly Lovers that featured interviews with dedicated spectrophiles.

The availability of zentai suits allows couples to at least act out the ghost rape fantasy. The woman struggles held by her lover clad head-to-toe in black. She is thrown to the bed or onto the floor. She writhes, terrified, in the grip of an unseen assailant who then, with adept caresses brings her to orgasm in his arms. In this fantasy, she may imagine that his actual appearance, which is concealed by his suit, is whatever she pleases. On the other hand, she knows nothing of his appearance. He might be the most handsome or the most ugly man in the world. She knows only she cannot help responding to him, cannot help yielding herself to her strong, invisible lover. She may set this fantasy, of course, in a larger context. Perhaps the ghost follows her about during the day. She does not know when he is with her and when he is not. Perhaps at her work, he whispers in her ear, startling and terrifying her, telling her that he will have her that evening. Perhaps when she is alone, she feels his hand at her waist, or on her breast, or leg, or maybe even her throat. Perhaps sometime he kisses her at the back of the neck. She can tell no one. They would think her insane. She is helpless, victimized. She hurries home, to rush within her apartment and lock the door. But he is waiting for her. Is he within the room or not? She does not know. She never knows. She prepares her bachelor-girl supper. She begins to be confident that she is alone. She feels safe. She becomes light hearted. She begins to sing. Then, suddenly, by unseen hands, she is gagged from behind. She is stripped, her hands are bound. She is then carried to the bed and thrown upon it. She is his for another night. He may have her much when he wishes. For example, she must fear, even in taking a shower or bath, for he might surprise her there, perhaps even taking her in the water. When she retires and steps naked to her closet to reach for her nightgown, perhaps he emerges from the closet, unseen, taking her frontally in his arms and smothering her cries with his kisses. He then warns her to silence and carries her, helpless, terrified, to her own bed.

For many, the novels of Ann Rice and more recently Twilight have created a fascination with vampires. Sometimes this can manifest itself as a yearning for a little edge play, although it turns out in most cases that the average person is not such a fan of blood in real life. Even so, the blood sucking lover is a huge turn on for many. Ever since Christopher Lee portrayed the Dracula as handsome Prince of Darkness in the early Hammer movies, the image of the blood sucking secret lover has been repeated over and over again. I personally knew a girl in university that bought a black Halloween cape with a red lining for her boyfriend and persuaded him to ravish her in a local church yard late at night. Actually I am not sure that he needed all that much persuading.

For a group of ravenous and villainous blood-sucking beasts, vampires have been remarkably glamourized, especially in the past ten years. The vampire has evolved from sexual predator to the object of sexual fantasy. TV series like Buffy and Twilight have created a whole generation of vampire fanatics, young women who spend hours drooling over specific characters and want nothing more than aggressive, frenetic sex with a blood sucker.

Vampires are portrayed with a deep, penetrating consciousness, whose full-hearted purpose leaves their lower impulses in the dust. Many ladies will openly admit that they want to be hunted. They fantasise about being spotted, zeroed in on, pursued, and claimed. For some this extends in the realms of being stalked, attacked and raped. For others it is much more romantic. They cannot resist a male whose deep care reaches further than his erection and can maintain that level of loving presence, even in the act of lovemaking. For many young women this is far more attractive, nourishing and honouring than a shallow ravenous impulse to get off. In many instances stories like True Blood have become forms of foreplay replacing the bodice-ripping, romantic fantasies of Barbara Cartland. Perhaps this is why vampire fiction is such a strong adolescent fantasy, because it is has such strong sexual overtones.

Sex is, on virtually all levels of existence, about power play. The male and the female are diametric opposites drawn together by an attraction which in many non-sexual environments simply does not exist. Most of us have at one time or another experienced lust or desire for someone we do not actually like as a person: it is the underlying reason why women fall for the 'bad guy'. And what more terrifying 'bad guy' exists than the vampire? In countless films the vampire has been portrayed as a sexual aggressor, his seduction being a means to an end just as it is with mortal men, except that the vampire's prime focus is blood not orgasm. But then look at the whole culture of female virginity as something so prized by men that they developed a religion utterly obsessed with it. What is this about if not blood? For many fang bangers, there is a strong element of S&M. Even in novels where the sex is unspoken, the aftermath speaks volumes. Sheets and pillows torn to shreds say it all. Vampire sex is rough.

Thanks to a boom in vampire fiction, there is a plethora of inspiration out there for those of you wishing to create your own vampire fantasies. The modern form of the genre begins with 'In Interview with a Vampire' the first of Anne Rice's Vampire Chronicles. Rice is the mother of all the modern Twilightesque novels, having pioneered the current generation of urban vampire stories. Many of the vampire books currently on the market are for Young Adults. If you are tired of all that teen angst in True Blood and want real vampire novels for adults where people act like adults (as opposed to whiny teenagers) here are some recommendations for some more X-rated versions. For a racy adult vampire series, Anita Blake, Vampire Hunter by Laurell K. Hamilton is as good a place as any to start. This series follows the exploits of a vampire hunter and raiser of zombies; it is a mix of fantasy, horror, and mystery genres. As the series develops the sexual themes become increasingly prominent. The combination of mystery and romance, has created a cult following of women who are turned on by vampire lovin'. The Dark-hunter Series by Sherrilyn Kenyon are so popular that they have even spawned a Manga series. These are atmospheric vampire romances with lots of sex, passion and action, and a reasonably interesting plot for good measure. The Black Dagger Brotherhood by J.R. Ward is a series about a group of vampires who defend their race and live in a highly sensual world. It is a character driven series that has won many awards and even more hearts. There is even a Vampire Seduction Handbook by Luc Richard Ballion and Scott Bowen. This is satirical step-by-step guide will help women the world over to experience the pleasures of vampire romance. It discusses balancing blood-play with physical thrills, and includes detailed descriptions of trysts across the ages.

Female vampires are always popular. We have even coined the term 'vamp' to describe this particular type of temptress. For some extreme inspiration, you might want to reasearch the Countess Alžbeta Bátoriová (Elizabeth Bathory) also known as the Blood Countess of Hungary. Born in 1560 in Nyírbátor, she was in life, one of the most notorious serial killers in Hungarian history, with detailed accounts in her own hand of how she killed 610 servant girls so that she could bathe in their blood.

Apart from the vampire, another common theme for the supernatural lover is that of the werewolf. This is perhaps one that is more difficult to pull off convincingly. There are now very realistic fursuits available on the market but they are still quite expensive. They are a far cry from the oversized mascots that we are used to seeing at football games and Disney parks, but at five hundred dollars for a quality example they might be a little out of reach for some couples. The Last Werewolf by Glen Duncan is a fantasy novel that is filled with lycanthropic sexual encounters but if you cannot find this then why not try to much more well known Little Red Riding Hood tale. All red outfits are simple to put together and most men enjoy playing the role of Big Bad Wolf.

The ghost role-playing scenario is particularly well suited to polyamorous threesomes, all of whom are lovers. One of the three players is a 'ghost,' invisible and inaudible to the other people. The two people who are not ghosts have a hot-n-heavy make-out session on the couch, while the ghost does whatever he or she likes to the other two people. The two people can not see or hear the ghost, but they can feel what the ghost does - so they blame the things on each other (for example, if the ghost gropes someone, that person will believe the other person did it). The ghost is free to do whatever he or she likes and touch or tease the others however he or she wants - completely blameless.

37. THE AFFAIR

The appealing thing about sex with complete strangers is the excitement of sex for sex's sake and the thrill of not knowing what you are going to get. Imagine you have gone to a bar and are sitting, having a cup of coffee or a drink, when your partner walks in and asks if she can share your table. Strike up a conversation. 'Do you come here often? What do you do with your free time? Do you have a partner or are you available?' Then let the conversation become more intimate. 'What sort of partner do you want and what sort of sex do you like?' Then she tells you she is feeling incredibly horny and is not wearing any panties. 'Want me to prove that to you?' she asks. You reply that you do, so she hitches up her skirt and asks whether what you see makes you hard. Then, even though you are supposed to be in a public place, she asks you to put your hand up her skirt, which you do. From here it is up to you whether to have sex there and then on the table or sneak to the toilet for sex with your new found friend. Best time to do this? How about just before she goes away for the weekend or you go away on business – that way you will not even have to spend the night with your 'stranger' after you have had sex. Add to the 'stranger' illusion by changing the way you look when you meet. Wear a suit if you usually wear jeans, get her to do her hair in a different style, and change your sexual technique or try things you would not normally do. This fantasy requires both of you to suspend your disbelief so you think you are in a public place and have just met. But how about meeting in a real café, having the same kind of conversation and then going for sex in a local hotel or even in your car if you can find a secluded place where you will not be caught? For inspiration, think about the spontaneous way you behaved with your partner when you first met.

The fantasy element here is, really, only that the lovers are unknown to one another. If she is going to have an affair, it might as well be with you. Why should you be left out? Similarly, if your boyfriend or husband is going to have an affair, why shouldn't it be with you? You can probably give him a better affair than some inexperienced, green youngster at the office who in all likelihood has not even been married yet. Such women, generally do not know one end of a man from the other. That takes a good deal of experience. Their concept of an affair is usually to lay down and have all their meals paid for.

The affair must be carefully planned. Ideally it takes place in a new locale, and, preferably, a rather exotic one. He may 'pick her up' in the bar, along the side walk, anywhere. Not all one-night stands begin at the bar or club. Somehow, it feels naughtier picking up your evening fling in the aisles of a book store, at the corner coffee shop or at a local art opening. Or maybe you meet each other for the first time at the hotel pool or by the ice machine – or in the elevator. Do not go over the top of course. Be polite to your fellow guests, not to mention the hotel staff. And keep things PG in public. He does not know her. But he is sexually interested in her. She is, to him, a new woman. Perhaps she has dyed her hair. She is now a blond, or a redhead, or a brunette. She is now something different. Moreover, she has purchased new clothes and new jewellery for this affair. He has never seen her dressed and adorned as he does now. Moreover she is probably 'his type.' They conduct themselves precisely as if they did not know one another. She plays coy. He tries tricks. They fence together verbally. He must be careful how he propositions her. She must be careful how she responds. The waiters, fellow guests, etc., do not know they are really a couple. He may have to make sure some other males do not 'cut in' on the woman he is after, etc. Only they know their real relationship. Both partners should talk to one another about themselves. When you are really interested in another person you wish to know a great many things about them, sometimes even small and intimate things. This is a time of relearning and re-appreciating one another, of reminding yourself of terribly important things you may have forgotten. This is a time to talk, and walk, and go dancing, and join one another in sight-seeing, and, in the evening, after supper, make love. Regardless,

207

chat each other up. Flatter your target. Flirt shamelessly. Make out in public. You can keep up the flirtation for as long as you like before you figure who is inviting who back to their room. Sometimes it is fun to pretend that you and your partner have not spent years getting to know each other's erotic ins and outs. What is more, you are not looking for a relationship – you are looking for quick and dirty sex, no bones about it. Tomorrow, you can be long time lovers again. Tonight, you are each other's one-night stand. Do not use your own first names. One-night-stand sex is purely physical, so take the opportunity to leave all your emotional baggage at home. Do not slip out of character and talk about family, job, or car troubles – real or fictional. Stick to small talk and enjoy your break from the everyday. You might even want to skip the romantic candlelit dinner entirely. You two can always go to brunch in the morning, once the scene is over and you are long-term lovers once again.

An interesting follow up to this is a scenario where you have placed an ad on a popular personals website seeking sexual escapades, no strings attached. Then you reserved your hotel room and waited for a hottie to take the bait. You stashed all your favourite toys in convenient berths by the bed, stripped down to something slinky, and now you are sitting by the phone. Someone calls. They have a nice voice. They start talking dirty. They start detailing exactly what they would like to do once they walk in the door. They have only one request – that you never ask their real name. You are on for a totally anonymous one-night encounter. Go wild.

38. The Captured

At the risk of being politically incorrect (something that is probably not worth worrying about in a book that deals openly with rape, bestiality and incest fantasies), I would like to suggest two classic scenarios, both of which have been dealt with extensively by the film industry and for which there is is plenty of celluloid inspiration. In the first section, the girl is captured by desert tribesmen while in the second she is abducted by red Indian braves.

Long before the current rise of Islamic fundamentalism, a movie entitled The Sheik starring Rudolph Valentino, was an enormous success, as was the sequel, Son of the Sheik. The books upon which the films were based were, in their time, were best sellers. It was not known, when it was published, that the author, E. M. Hull was a woman and it caused something of a stir when it leaked out. Doubtless much of the success of the movies was due to the remarkable performances of the late, great Valentino. Few other actors then or since have been able to express such joy in touching a woman as well as he. On the screen Valentino conveyed that women are marvellously desirable and beautiful creatures. Valentino could portray the looming, dark, male menace, dangerous, desirable, sensuous, intent upon her sexual subjugation, but, too, like perhaps no other actor, he could, when he wished, exhibit that he was almost uncontrollably thrilled and delighted to hold a woman in his arms. If that is flattery, it is flattery that will get a man just about anywhere.

His was a more romantic generation. Cloak swirling, on his Arabian stallion, he bore her with him, a captive, to his tent in the desert, there to be ravished at his leisure. Women, in his day, pale, proud and beautiful, were thought to be worthy prizes, worth capturing and carrying off. Valentino realized and create something which could be accepted as an authentic fantasy dream, of many women. For those used to the CGI of modern blockbusters, silent movies may seem dated and even dull but actually, they are simply a different version of the same art form, in just the same way that modern art is different to renaissance portraiture. Both are appreciated in different ways. The movies of the silent era can be wonderful inspiration for sexual fantasy. For women, I recommend the films of Louise Brooks whose facial expressions can turn from innocent coquette to brazen harlot in milliseconds.

There are elements in the desert fantasy which make it exotic and intoxicating. The desert, with its oases, caravans, camel bells, dancing girls, striped tents, palm trees and bandits, remains a romantic locale. It certainly beats down-town Ipswich or mid-western Idaho. Furthermore, the position of the woman in Arabian culture, particularly in the past, was very low. Thus if an aristocratic English lady, for example, were captured, she would have been thrust into a very uncomfortable position, which in some ways makes the fantasy all the more delicious. To begin with she is only a female; furthermore she is a captive. Worse still she is an infidel, a cultural 'outsider' worthy of little or no respect. She is less than an animal, completely at their mercy. She is also a woman of the enemy. It is only to be expected that their hatred of the west, which threatens their way of life, and regards itself as superior to them will make itself evident. Their rage and resentment, will be vented upon her. They will make the West pay and she will stand proxy for the West. We can expect that she will be put to repeated and harsh abuse. She is their secret prisoner; no one knows her whereabouts; she cannot escape across the desert; she is helplessly theirs. Dressed revealingly for their tactile and visual pleasures, she can now be bought and sold; she must be obedient; she must do whatever she is told; she is now only an educated, white slave girl, the property of her Arab masters. What happens to her, what is done to her, is up to the creators of the fantasy.

In the western frontier version of this fantasy, she is captured by marauding Indian warriors. If you have the opportunity to enjoy horseback riding you can play parts of this as you are out riding. It also works well if you are hikers or campers, where the openness of nature, with its fresh air and stimulating scenery can provide an incomparable setting for the fantasy's enactment. See chapter 24 for more information regarding the joys of camping sex. How many men have had the chance to actually pursue their wife through a woods, or among hills, and then to have captured her? Girls love running from a man they would be delighted to be caught by. It seems to be in their blood both to flee and to yield deliciously, delightedly, when, inevitably, they fall prey. The chase is, probably for genetic reasons going back to evolutional selections, sexually stimulating to them; it is, of course, disappointing to them if, at its conclusion, they are not captured, and, uncompromisingly, sexually possessed by their captor.

If you wish, she may be given a short head start, say, some ten or fifteen minutes before trailing her. Make sure that she leaves a reasonable trail to follow or you could both end up wandering lost in the bush. This fantasy should not be enacted in nature if there is any danger of the partners becoming lost.

A tent, with its privacy, can serve well enough for a teepee or wigwam. A small camp can serve as the encampment of a brave with his prize, a captured white woman. Indians often found more of interest in white women than their hair. It was not unknown for them to be carried off and used as slaves. Their position in the Indian camp was miserable. They were lower than squaws and squaws hated them, and could beat them with sticks to make them do their work. In the teepee they were only a despised woman of another race, a female of the enemy.

Furthermore she stood outside the family and friendship ties of the camp. An Indian girl of one's own tribe would always be the daughter of another warrior. The white captive does not share the same standing. What does the tribe care what he does to her? The more he abuses her and the more harshly he treats her, the more they will be pleased. The lot of the white slave girl of an Indian master would not be an easy one. She would well learn what it would be to be a simple female at the mercy of men. She would learn it in the camp and, at night, she would learn it in the teepee of her master. A blanket may be thrown over her head and, by means of a belt, tied about her belly. This is based on an authentic American Indian technique for keeping a white slave woman quiet. When the slave cannot see, she tends to become docile, one which is also effective of livestock.

In the bedroom with you in the next room, the woman can always be 'abandoned' for fifteen minutes or so, to permit her to struggle with her bonds, understand herself helpless and build up suspense. When you return to her then, you can pretend that she has been tied 'for hours,' helplessly, waiting for you to return to her, and have your will with her. During this time, these many hours, she has not known what her fate was to be. When you return to her, she is bound as perfectly, as securely, as when you left her. She looks at you with terror. She knows that she is yours. What will you do with her?

This fantasy, of course, need not be enacted outdoors. It, like any other, can be happily enacted in the bedroom. Indeed, it can be experimented with, and developed, in the bedroom and then, later, if the partners wish, taken outdoors. It may, of course, happily remain, too, in the bedroom, which can be, to the lovers, a thousand different worlds. Nor do you need to restrict yourselves to these two scenarios alone. The captive fantasy lends itself to almost any historical period. You might imagine yourself as the Scarlet Pimpernel rescuing a French aristocrat from certain death. The hitch hiker abducted by a dissolute pack of Hells Angels. The Mayan princess enslaved by the evil conquistadors. The peasant girl taken by a band of devil worshipping monks. The possible combinations are endless.

39. The Job Interview

S eated before a prospective employer – a man in a suit, in a high rise building the woman finds herself in an unfortunate predicament. She needs this job desperately and is forced, against her will, to try to buy what she needs with her flesh. The male, callous, in a commanding position, imposes his demands. She does not have to accept his demands. It is only that if she does not, she will not get the job. If she does make the sacrifice, she might get the job. Then again, she might not. Many women, unfortunately find themselves in such positions, especially in Asian cultures, where it is not unknown for female advancement and promotion to depend on her sexual prowess. Whereas a situation of this sort, in real life, is an ugly and unpleasant one, in fantasy, it can sometimes provide pleasure for a woman. It has something of the 'whore' element going for it, except that the woman performs under 'duress.' She must, nonetheless, perform. It is a form of 'forced sex' and forced sex is a frequently encountered element in sexual fantasy. A tinge of shame and helplessness, if a part of the game, can be sexually delicious. In the motion picture industry this is also known as the casting couch fantasy.

Many women confess that their fantasies are far more intricate than a simple interview situation. Here for example a poster from one the more popular forums confesses a much more demanding scenario:

"I fantasise that I'm in a job interview and that I have to strip to my underwear in front of the panel of three men. They ask me intimate questions about my sexual preferences while I'm made to stand before them. On the table is an assortment of sex toys which of which I'm expected to chose from and then demonstrate the use of for them."

Perhaps even more exciting than the job interview is the disciplinary interview. Here is an interesting example of how it could play out if you so wished. This has been excerpted from a popular spanko gathering site.

Technically there were lots of options. She could take the reprimand on her file. She could change departments, accept a reassignment. She could resign. With the blot on her record she would not even be able to get a job as a ditch digger, but she had choices. Not good ones, but they were there.

In reality, of course, there were no choices and they both knew it. Her entire future was dependent upon what happened in this room in the next few minutes. Nearly a decade of her life, years of academic study, ruthless devotion to physical fitness, and endless training in a variety of fields was all about to be washed down the drain.

He had placed the high-backed chair in the middle in his office. The other employees had already left for the day, so they had sufficient privacy. 'When you're working for me and I have to discipline you again, it will happen after hours like today, the other employees don't need to know about it." She blushed when she realized he had already decided this would not be a one time thing.

"Whatever number you're thinking of, double it," he said sternly. "This must be 'strict'. I cannot allow subordinates to think they can get away with screw ups scot-free."

"I'll punish you when you're disrespectful." He said. 'But there are other reasons that could warrant punishment as well. I already mentioned an unhappy customer, but showing up late and failing to meet a deadline will also earn you a trip to my office. Understood young lady?" His voice had changed slightly, he was in control now and she a naughty girl being reprimanded. When she confirmed she understood he told her to lift her bottom. His hands reached below her and unzipped her pants. She blushed when he pulled them down. Her bottom was glistening in sweat after his warm hands' rubbing, her panties sticking against her cheeks leaving nothing to the imagination. But he did not even leave her that little bit of covering. He told her all punishment should be administered on bare flesh, and even though she protested he pulled down her panties as well. Completely exposed to him she should not feel surprised to feel embarrassment. But it was not her nudity that embarrassed her that much, it was more a source

214

of excitement. She felt embarrassed for getting punished like a little girl, already embarrassed for the reason for this spanking as if she was already learning a lesson on good behaviour. And thinking that made her blush even more, she had never thought of herself as someone who needed lessons in good behaviour.

"I'm not a bad girl that needs to be punished," She thought to herself "I'm a good girl that wants to be taught a lesson."

The first stroke came as a surprise. She had still been thinking about her feelings, but was roughly reminded of her current situation by the stinging pain in her left cheek. The rod hissed in warning like a snake before it kissed her tender behind. It seemed he was not going to be gentle with her and although it was not severe, the strokes came quicker than the pain could subdue and the stinging rose to a hot and burning feeling. All thoughts of embarrassment vanished and all she could think of was her aching bottom.

It was not the erotic situation she had imagined in her dreams, it was more real, a real beating for a naughty girl, meant to hurt and teach her a lesson. And yet somehow that turned her on even more than those in her dreams had. Tears formed in the corners of her eyes and she squealed and yelped at every stroke. But her hips made a rocking motion against his lap, in time with his movements. She was not sure she was doing that to in an attempt to escape the punishment or to rub against the bulge in his pants. Thoughts about the wet spot between her legs eventually vanished as well however when the session reached its peak. The only thought that remained was embarrassment for her behaviour and truly feeling sorry for what she had done. Her bottom burned and she kicked her legs trying to shake off the feeling. She told him she had learned her lesson, begged him to stop, cried out, tears rolling down her cheeks, ruining her make-up.

He made a point of not stopping until she stopped begging, as if proving to her that he stopped when he wanted to, not when she asked. She lay sobbing across his lap and his hand softly caressed her bare red bottom. "I'm sorry I had to be so hard on you." He said "But I had to make sure you realized from the start the this punishment meant something, that I really mean them to teach you something and not just a sexual fantasy I want to use you for."

He let her catch her breath after his short explanation, his hand silently stroking her bottom. She did not want to talk, she just wanted to lay there and enjoy his hand on her bottom. But she realized her silence might make him feel uncomfortable. 'That's good,' she said. 'If they weren't real, I might misbehave on purpose, and that would be bad for business.' She blushed as she realized she meant that. She felt 'better' somehow, after this experience.

His hand squeezed her bottom more roughly after she said that and she could not suppress a soft moan. 'I knew there was a moment you were enjoying it a bit too much,' he said.

His hand was caressing her sore bottom more roughly now and she bit her lip, it hurt, but she could not stop herself from making that rocking movement again, rubbing against that bulge that proved she was not the only one that enjoyed it too much. 'Maybe you know some remedy for that as well.' She asked.

'I do.' He answered. 'But that would be inappropriate in a work-relationship, unless you would enjoy dinner tonight?' She answered his question by a long low moan. 'Good, I'll pick the restaurant, one with good hard wooden chairs, I want to see you squirm.'

'Anything you say.' She replied in a blush as his hand squeezed her sore bottom.

'Just don't think this means I'll be light on you next time.' He said.

'I wouldn't want you to…

40. The Mating Pouch

If you were wondering what what you could do with that sleeping bag while you are not away camping, then here is a interesting fantasy that takes advantage of a very exciting environment. Of course you can also try this out when you are out sleeping under the stars.

Two Earthling slaves, a beautiful woman and a strong handsome man, prisoners of an alien race, are placed naked in a mating pouch. Many sleeping bags are so designed that two can be zipped together. This produces a bag that is twice the size of a normal bag. It can be great fun to make love for change under such confining conditions and it is a very different and sensuous experience.

For background, imagine that you are two earthlings that have managed to escape their alien overlords. After a long and exhausting pursuit through the exotic flora of the alien's planet, the pair are recaptured. They had originally selected for the mating pouch but had attempted to resist the procedure. Even though they had been chosen with great technological precision out of a huge population they had decided to rebel against the wishes of their captors. Extensive scientific tests had shown conclusively that they were an ideal match. They were perfect mates, because they would be totally and irresistibly attracted to one another. If it were not for the aliens, who, of course, are interested only in breeding animals, they would never have found one another. Rather than be subjected to the ignominious breeding program they decided to make a bolt for freedom. Unfortunately, their escape did not last long and now they are back in the breeding facility. The man and woman are helpless to resist the flood tides of their instincts, have no choice but to mate.

In order to add more colour to this scenario imagine that the slaves have no names, only identification numbers.

"I am earth female specimen 33782."

"I am earth male specimen 66715."

The aliens keep Earthlings in mated slave pairs as the aggressive males are easier to control when an attractive female given to them as their mate (is this not the way males are controlled on our own planet?) If he is disobedient or recalcitrant, she is taken from him, and given to another slave. She might be exchanged for a less desirable mate, or he might be deprived of a female entirely. There are many different possibilities.

Another option is to have the lovers chained together at the waist. Each wears a belt through which the chain passes. This keeps the lovers in proximity, facing one another, and gives them enough room to hold and touch one another. Alternatively, they might be attached by the wrists. If you both have collars then being joined at the throat is a deliciously sensuous sensation.

41. The Oldest Profession

Across the globe, there are many classes of brothels. Slavery is banned in most places, but not all and this represents some of the most barbaric establishments. South East Asian chicken shacks where the girls are kept in the pitch dark and customers pay to run wild inside, doing whatever they want to whomever they please are perhaps the lowest of the low. Dirty, low-class flop-houses with uneducated floozies are a slight step up the ladder but not far. Slightly more civilised institutions are the most prevalent in the western world at the moment. These range from the mustang ranches of Nevada to the legalised brothels of Australia. Finally there are the high-class (read extortionately expensive) establishments where the wealthy, the powerful and the privileged indulge their secret fantasies. Some of the more famous examples might include the Hollywood mansion of Madam extraordinaire Heidi Fleiss or the opulent sex palaces of Buenos Aires. There are even the thinly disguised but incredibly expensive karaoke parlours in Lhasa, Tibet which cater to the free-spending, high-ranking officers of the Chinese Red Army occupiers. At the other end of the nation are the infamous saunas and massage parlours of Dongguan, where vast sexual menus are designed to tempt millionaire Chinese industrialists. Most of the services available are written as wildly esoteric Chinese idioms that reveal little about the true salacious nature of the 'service' itself. Factory owner clients who think nothing of spending a thousand dollars in a single evening are treated like living gods. Many of the menu items sound like secret martial-arts techniques and include the following:

Roaming the Wide World – A slow tongue bath of the entire body

Desert Storm – A blow-job with pop rocks

Cleansing the Dragon Gate – A manual washing and stimulating the the anus

Flowing Water, Golden Mountain – Sweeping the entire body with a mouthful of water

Ice and Fire; Nine Steps to Heaven – A blow-job with alternating mouthfuls of ice and hot water

Seeking the Moon Under the Sea – Delicately biting and nibbling the testicles

Roaming the North Pole – An ice water tongue bath

Countless Ties and a Thousand Links – Using long hair tresses to tickle and stimulate the body

Ten Fingers Linked to the Heart – Pulling ten fingers until a popping sound is heard for each digit

Other more esoteric practises include the wild cat frenzy, the monkey stealing peaches, toppling the mountains and overturning the seas, the jade hand Goddess of Mercy and sweet dew oozing from the heart. Not being a member of the Chinese nouveau riche, I am quite not sure what these are referring to to but I have included them here in case you wish to add them to your own personal fantasies.

Using the the oldest profession as the basis of a sexual fantasy can be extremely exciting. Here the man actually pays for his partner's services and accordingly, treats her as the whore she is. She, on the other hand, acts like a real whore in the bedroom. There is a little bit of whore in every woman and prostitution is a common fantasy for many. Every woman is probably curious to know if she could make her living, and how successfully, by her body. Actual prostitution, with its haste, its degradation, its diseases, its commercialism, is an ugly and unfortunate business. On the other hand, as play, between loving partners, it can be very enjoyable.

Treating a women as 'the whore she is' is meant in the context of the fantasy. Even so, for many western men with no direct experience of prostitution this can be a challenge. Firstly, it is important not to be truly callous with her, nor hurt her feelings. You are both playing. If you treat her callously, it will not be much fun for her. If you play "treating her callously" it can be delicious for her. Even if she were a real life prostitute, there is no excuse in the world for treating her callously. Even the genuine whore is a human being and deserves the same consideration and affection accorded to any other person. These girls are forced through dire economic circumstance to provide sexual services and should be treated with affection and respect.

On the other hand, in the fantasy, a whore may be treated with a certain degree of objective bluntness. In particular, since you are paying for her, you want quality performance. If she wants her tricks to come back, if she wants to stay in business, she had better be good. Tell her what you want done, and how you want it done, if necessary. You are paying her. You make her work for you. Make her sweat a little to please you. Lay there and make her work for her money.

The matter of payment is of interest. I suggest that you pay her with real money. A couple of genuine bills placed under her body where she can feel them, might be appropriate. She will not object, perhaps to your surprise, at earning the money for a new handbag in this fashion. Your partner is, after all, like any other woman, deliciously, part whore. She should certainly not be expected to return the money to you. Why should she? The poor girl has worked for it, and earned it.

A interesting variant here is the 'French Whore' fantasy. If your partner speaks French, so much the better. If not, it does not matter. In this version, she is paid in French money. In this case you will probably wish to use the same currency again and again. If she feels cheated, of course, you can, later, give her the local currency equivalent. It is important to maintain good international relations. Probably, for this fantasy, she should locate some of that scandalously shocking, charming black lingerie. Garter belt, dark stockings, black choker, etc., are all very appropriate. You are familiar, doubtless, with the picture, one that provides a delightfully stimulating fantasy. Even something like a French magazine opened on the dresser, or a French CD playing in the background can add interesting and stimulating detail.

Another variant is that in which the locale is somewhat more exotic. Perhaps the male partner is on shore leave in Zanzibar. He is a rough sailor, on leave from his ship. He wants some fun. What sort of woman is it who awaits him? Does she wear a veil? Did she, below, on the first floor, belly dance for him while he ate, only then, when he signified his interest, to be sent upstairs by the proprietor of the establishment to wait for him? Is she a native woman, or is she a western woman, who, because of debts or known secrets, is at the mercy of the owner of the establishment? Is she a woman who has been conditioned to the mastery of men, or is she that western woman who, in fear of the power of the owner of the establishment, is forced to be more delightful and more servile than any native girl could dream of being?

For a Victorian steam-punk variation on this theme, I like the stories of the notorious pixie named Nel, also known as Dirty Nellie to human occult researchers. Nel is Street Faerie prostitute often working in the theatre district of London. She got her start at the dawn of the Victorian age as a simple street walker. She would use her supernatural powers to appear as whatever she felt her clients were looking for. Her most oft used guise is that of a coster girl who has lost all her snells and needs to make back all her lost money or her cruel stepfather will beat her. She has also been known to appear as dusky beauty from the orient, or a young lad lost in the city after leaving his boarding school.

Though guile, deceit and lots of hard work, Nel worked her way into the prominent occult societies of the time. As her clientele increased in wealth and status, so did her own. She gained not only monetary wealth, but a wealth of information about such organizations as the Algernon Club, the Rosicrucians, the Hermetic Order of the Golden Dawn (where she was Aleister Crowley's lover for a time), and the Theosophical Society.

Role playing Dirty Nellie is great fun because she is the archetypical good-time girl. When not working she can be found in gambling houses, public houses, or even an opium den. Her looks in any form are striking. She is vain and proud of her looks, her midnight black hair (cut short) and her green eyes. She is fond of soldiers and once travelled to India to be with an entire troupe. She returned to London with a pierced nose and an addiction to the bindi cigarettes smoked there. Her favourite trick is to produce one she has pre-rolled from nowhere and light it with the tip of her finger. As a Faerie, Nel is immune to the harmful effects of her addictions to smoking, alcohol and drugs, as well as the other afflictions that plague her trade. Nel is not a fighter but she is not above threatening someone with her knife. Nel would rather seduce someone and then poison them in the bed chamber if she wants someone dead. Usually though trouble finds Nel and not the other way around. A possible introduction would be having her running for her life and smack right into the male parter, playing the Victorian gentleman in the Professor Higgins role. The musical My Fair Lady is a wonderful source of inspiration for this fantasy.

Despite some of her addictions, arrogance and her rather rude habit of calling humans monkeys, Nel is actually a very sweet faerie girl. She is also just determined to do things her way. One thing is certain, it is never boring with her around. Her clothing is usually a motley assortment that revealed more flesh than even the most brazen dolly-mop would have been shamed to show. If you approach her for a closer inspection, her first reaction might be along the lines of, "Oi! Piss off. I'm trying to work 'ere!"

For a more contemporary setting, high-end hotels are home to much more than business travellers charging room service to their company's credit card. It may be illegal, but everyone knows that escorts routinely use hotels to conduct their business. In the call-girl fantasy, you have placed your call and your paid companion for the evening has agreed to meet you in the hotel bar. She tells you what she will be wearing – some signature item such as a pair of red high heels, a scarf around her neck, or maybe a distinctive brooch on her lapel.

Take advantage of the hotel ambience to indulge in a little harmless but hot fantasy play. Many escorts wear business suits to their out-call appointments, with extra-sexy lingerie hidden underneath. But if you would rather use this scenario as an excuse to don your trashiest outfit and make-up, go for it. Do not forget to pack a gear bag, too. Stash spare lingerie, lube, toys and any other 'extras' you might want. Buy her a drink and make some small talk before heading to your hotel room. She can perform a strip tease down to her lingerie to warm up, then strip you down to your underwear and provide a lap dance. After that, negotiations for specific services can begin. Do not be shy. Ask for exactly what you want. Remember, she is a pro. Keep the focus on purely sexual satisfaction. It is also fun to make up a fake working name to go with your prostitute persona. Porn star, stripper and white trash names include Angel, Brandy, Candy, Honey, Jade, Roxy and Tiffany, but here are few others that you might want to try.

Lucy Lips
Fonda Cox
Peaches LaTour
Cupcakes Cassidy
Anita S. Pankin.
Ling Ling Rodriguez
Mona Cummings
Cherry Hardwood
Bonanza Ryder
Ferocia Coutura
Pussy Galore
Summer Swallows
Peach Bottoms
Summer Swallows
Felicity Shagswell

As an interesting aside, the Brunching Shuttlecocks website has an interesting online quiz entitled 'Porn Star or My Little Pony?'
Can you tell the difference between the names that are given to a very popular children's toy and those that have been chosen by hardcore sex actors. You might be surprised how difficult this innocuous looking test turns out to be.

brunching.com/pornorpony.html

Maybe you do not want a full-service encounter. You just want some tender loving touch from a pretty girl or handsome lad. Strip the blankets off the bed and lay some towels down. Put a bottle of massage oil on the night stand. Take off your clothes, put on a robe, and call your partner. He or she will play the role of sensual masseuse. All you have to do is lie back and enjoy yourself while your masseuse explores every inch of your body, from the crown of your head to the toes on your feet. Encourage your masseuse to take off their clothes, too, and rub you down with their chest, thighs, hair, or whatever other body part they choose to use. Make it a full-contact experience. And yes, make sure to give your client the proverbial happy ending.

Remember that not all prostitutes are female. From the rent-a-rastas that ply their trade on the beaches of Montego Bay to the outrageously expensive pretty-boy hosts of Tokyo's Shinjuku and Shibuya districts, there are a wide range of gigolos in the twenty first century. Their job is to fulfil a lady client's every wish. Whatever she asks for – her wish is his command. The session can start with a sensual striptease, down to briefs or g-string. Or he could offer to give her a sensual massage. Whatever comes next, what is certain is that her pleasure is top priority. Pack a vibrator and plenty of toys in your kit. Talk dirty and shower her with compliments. But let her call the shots all night long. You do not get off until she is completely satisfied. She is sure to tip big when the time comes. Remember that male prostitute names are even wilder than their female counterparts. Here are a few suggestions.

Lance Thruster
Rod Longstaff
Luke Thighwalker
Spike Bighorn
Eric von Pumpaloaf
Blade Steel
Harry Plowman
Dr. Barry McKockiner
Emerson Biggins
Chet Swinghard
Holden McGroyne
Biff Lungewright

Damien Cashmere
Craven Morehead
Rider Strong
Jimmy Everhard
Maximus Johnson
Shaft Longley
Harry Balzania
Max Thrust
Myles O'Toole
Harden Long
Doug Thumper
Brady Afterburn
Willy Fisterbottom
Jack Hammer
Colt Steel
Stanley Giggledick
Lance Hardwood
Sterling Archer
Harry Danglebag
Rusty Springs
Dick McIroncock
Hans Downerpants
Wolfgang Longsocks
Willard Midnight
And if you are a visiting Nollywood Porn star, try Mustaffa Mehrod Enjapuper.

43. The Pet Fantasy

For extreme fantasy lovers, imagine a planet in a distant galaxy which is home to the headquarters of huge intergalactic company, manned by aliens, specializing in what is, in effect, a display and pet industry. Here on earth, many of us are very fond of such things as dogs and cats. For others this extends exotic flora and aquaria of tropical fish, etc. We like to have such things in our home and we might also suppose that other forms of rational life have similar interests in such activities. A high-order form of alien life, for example, might find it decorative for its residence to be adorned with certain forms of life as pets. Perhaps some of these forms of alien life are several feet tall, or weigh many tons, so that their physical relation to humans would be approximately that of ours to puppies and kittens.

In these great shops various plants and pets from across the galaxy are available for pet connoisseurs. A terrarium of purple Neptunian ice lichens. A pair of sand skittlers from Venus, with appropriate gases for its tank; a floppy eared six-legged bunglebaby from Hephaestus II; an oversized sloth-like phleme from the equatorial highlands of Titian 14. Most interestingly we also find a young, shapely, two-legged, long-haired Earth female, from the temperate grasslands of the planet Earth, an interesting, bluish, watery planet on the borders of civilization.

Such specimens are caught (trapped, netted, hooded) with no more thought than the snaring of any other sort of animal, for which there is a price. The bounty hunters, hired by aliens, are organized and efficient. Earth, a backward nation, lies much at the mercy of these depredations. The females are treated with the same efficiency and care as any other form of desired commercial animal. They are caught, rounded up, herded, stripped, kept in holding areas, fed and watered, examined as to condition and health, graded and sorted, etc. If found acceptable for return to the alien's planet, they might be branded with the company's mark; each is doubtless provided with a locked collar, perhaps with ring for leash attachment, coded to inform purchasers of her approximate age, place and time of capture, grade, health data, diet, etc. The age is estimated primarily by size, development of female contours, general appearance, dryness of hair and condition of teeth. In examining the teeth, the head is forced back and the mouth opened rudely with two hands, holding the jaws apart. This serves to open the mouth widely and, as a precautionary measure, prevents biting. Captured Earth females, on the other hand, to the interest of the hunters, almost never bite. Only one in ten thousand attempts to bite. She, of course, is promptly punished, usually by a severe whipping. She will not attempt to bite again. She has learned obedience under the lash, and well. She will now be even more eager to please than the others. The rest are too terrified. They wish only to obey and be pleasing. Earth females are prize slave stock, highly valued in the galaxy. A touch of the whip turns any one of them into a superb slave.

On the alien planet, and where the company maintains its outlets, the girls are available for purchase by various forms of rational life, including wealthy Earthlings. One beauty might find herself purchased by a large, slug-like creature, who keeps her in his globe, as an olfactory ornament, pleased by her smells. Another is kept as a part of a collection of interesting and diverse fauna, used primarily as educational tool. A third finds herself introduced into a distant household as a lovely pet by two childless aliens who take her for walks on a lead. Others are purchased, in large groups, for scientific experiments, which the aliens would regard as immoral to inflict on individuals of their own type; such specimens are kept in heavy wired cages, with metal plates.

Earthlings rich enough and well enough placed in the commercial unions of the galaxy, may well frequent such shops. We might imagine ourselves as a visiting Federation diplomat, perhaps we make a purchase on impulse. A cute little captive literally begs us to buy her. Or maybe you are an intergalactic trader, with your own star ship dropping off a consignment of wookie furs, and are now interested in picking up a female of your own kind. After many months of trapping and hunting you are rough and you smell of matted fur. The beauty in the cage is highly intelligent, sensitive, well-educated, a most aristocratic woman. You can tell from her gaze that she is a proud, spoiled beauty, that she has never been beaten. Moreover you see that she has lost the initial fears of the captive girl, the terror and shock commonly attendant on their taking by the slavers; she has now regained something of her pride and insolence; perhaps she dares to tell you, "Do not look at me!"; perhaps she comes, arrogantly, to the bars and poses before you, "Do you like what you see?"; you can tell that she despises you, that she loathes you as an ill-educated boor, a ruffian; you buy her anyway. You immediately put her in steel restraints. Turning her sharply about, you snap the metal device about her midriff, putting your arms around her, locking it shut in front. You thrust her wrists into the attached metal claspers, snapping them closed and locking them. She glares at you in fury. Once secured you seize her by the hair and kiss her roughly. You have been alone in space for months. She, similarly sex starved since her capture, is visibly shaken, as a female. "I hate you!" she says. She might view you as dirty, loathsome and contemptible, but at the same time she is frightened. She sees you as a powerful male in whose very presence she feels aroused, fighting the feeling, hating herself for it, weak and submissive. You hook your leash, a light metal one, through which the animal cannot chew, on her collar, and lead her on this tether, your purchased pet, to your ship.

"I hate you!" she cries.

"I hate you!" You smile. You have had this experience with other women. You know this beauty will yield to you in the end, tears in her eyes, crying out to you her slavery.

"You will never tame me," she says.

To herself she fantasizes yielding to you, as a helpless slave girl. She feels very receptive, very feminine, very weak. When he reaches the ship he puts his hand on her. She is already wet, liquid and hot. He holds his hand before her face. "I know," she says. She turns her head away, refusing to look at him. He locks her leash to a steel step of the ship, and climbs the stairs to the navigation room, saving the breaking in process for later. You touch the door switch and the two steel doors, forming the lock, slide shut, closing her inside.

44. THE SLAVE AUCTION

Some women are intensely curious to learn what price their flesh would bring at auction. Society encourages a woman to see herself as an object of desire. They wonder what it would be like to be stripped and placed on the auction block of a slave market for the examination of buyers. They wonder what it would be like to have men bidding for their body. What would they sell for? This fantasy gives them an opportunity to find out.

Not all women are born as slaves. Some might be kidnapped tourists, a beautiful female tourist who finds herself captured and placed in such a market. Another variant could be the young female journalist intent on doing an exposé of the slave trade. She bribes her way into highly secretive auction house disguised as a local with her camera and her notebooks concealed beneath her robe. This will be a major 'scoop' and will make a fantastic front page story. She discovers, for example, that white women as well as blacks are sold in this particular auction house.

Unbeknownst to her she has been tricked. Once she has obtained her pictures and her story and is ready to leave, the net closes in. There is a pre-arranged signal and she is revealed to the assembled buyers as a western intruder. With a whip she is driven to the block and stripped. As she is forced to remove her clothing, the bids increase, article by article. Eventually she is sold, and her buyer, binding and gagging her, takes her home.

Not all women are keen to feel the lick of a whip. Not everybody enjoys that kind of sensation. If you are unsure about your partners penchant for pain then I suggest that you simply, sharply, clap your hands, and the woman reacts as though struck. The beating is therefore completely symbolic and fantasy is fantasy. Moving her body as though it were under the whip of a man can give women pleasure; and, too, pretending to strike them, and seeing her react as if struck, can produce

231

an incredible sense of dominance in a male. If she cannot see when your hands strike together the movement of her body, startled, will be extremely realistic. Your "blows" should be timed in such a way that different intervals obtain between them. She should not know when the "blow" is coming. She must wait for it, tense, frightened. Then, when it does fall, she reacts, startled, piteously, as though actually struck, as though feeling great pain. One way of achieving an interesting effect is to tie her naked, on her stomach, on the bed, her wrists and ankles tied apart to the bed posts, with a pillow inserted between her legs and under her body. This way, when she writhes, she will be stimulated by her movements against the pillow. This combines the psychological gratification, common in female fantasies, of being completely at the mercy of a dominant male, with the intimate physiological stimulation, as though she were helpless to prevent it, two delights often combined in female sexual fantasy.

There are many different males roles here that can be acted out. Perhaps she is kept for a time before she is sold and therefore requires a keeper. How is she restrained? Is she chained in her cell? Does he shackle her? What is she fed? Is she permitted to use her hands to feed herself? Must she kneel to eat out of a dish with her mouth, her hands tied behind her? Does the keeper feed her by hand? Does he throw her scraps of food, like a dog? A second male role is that of the auctioneer. Doubtless she is expected to perform well on the block. Doubtless she is expected to excite the interest of the buyers? Does her auctioneer, on the block, caress her intimately, so that the buyers may see that the slave is sexually responsive? Finally there is the role of the buyer who eventually purchases the slave and takes her home.

The sales of such slaves may be public or private. Perhaps the human livestock is privately exhibited only to certain selected buyers, just one at a time? And perhaps each of these buyers is entitled to try out the quality of the goods being inspected. Public sales (in which there are many buyers) or private (in which there are few buyers, or only one) may be detailed and exquisite, or swift and rude. Different scenarios provide differing levels of stimulation to different women.

To be sold before many men is almost a ritual of commerce. At the other end of the scale, to be summarily disposed of for a quickly agreed-upon price to a single buyer is a very different experience. In a 'quick-sale' situation, the woman, nude, and bound hand and foot, is thrown to the feet of a prospective buyer to be rapidly assessed and bid upon. Perhaps he caresses her to note her responsiveness. She will probably writhe helplessly, her bonds creating a delicious agony of shame and sexual stimulation. Not all societies are as financially sophisticated as that of the West in the twenty first century. Some more primitive cultures might still be in the habit of bartering for goods. How would your woman react if you traded her for camels or goats? Perhaps you could emphasise the rarity of her alabaster white skin and trade her for a dozen jungle females of which the chief has a vast surplus. The barter concept leads to some very interesting story lines.

An intergalactic exploration mission is crewed by five internationally renowned scientists, four men and one woman, all leaders in their fields of expertise. Due to massive instrument failure, the vessel deviates considerably from course and, eventually, crashes on a small, uncharted planet, one of thousands in this unknown galaxy. Despite their doctorates in computer science, exo-biology and astrophysics they are ill prepared for what comes next.

Only a few days after crash landing, the scientists are visited by the local inhabitants. The natives of this new world are familiarly humanoid and there are five of them. Four are huge barbarian warriors, almost the complete opposite of the eggheads that make up the earthling astronauts. The fifth is an an exquisite, excitingly clad female, collared and branded, who serves the barbarian freebooters as a slave.

Lost and helpless on this strange new world, the humans are in dire need of the aliens' assistance. Communication, by gestures and words, is managed. The aliens' visit is accompanied by gifts of heady wine and local delicacies. The beautiful alien slave girl serves all of food and drink. She is beautiful and submissive, and very concerned to be pleasing. The Earth men are stunned with the unexpected pleasure of being treated by a woman as though they might be important. This is very different to their own female colleague, Dr. Vivian Stephenson, a prim and proper palaeo-anthropologist who is far more concerned with her research than any male-to-female interaction. The alien beauty is by comparison in awe of the earthmen, if only because they are free men. She herself is only a lowly female slave. This in turn sets of an unexpected chain reaction. Suddenly, as never before, unusual emotions, primitive emotions, flood the veins of the scientists. Their blood is suddenly aware, as it never was on their own world, of their masculinity. It seems that on this world women are kept as animals and slaves. It is a decision they had made, long ago, as men. There is immediate friction, of course, between the lovely slave and the straight laced anthropologist in her asexual jumpsuit and androgynous crew cut. This is to be expected. They are two very different conceptions of female. The slave, in the presence of the human female feels her servitude much more cruelly. Dr Stephenson in turn, resents the slave's obvious attractions to the male crew members, and treats her with unnecessary harshness.

On the other hand, the leader of the barbarians does not fail to recognize that the scientist is a female of the species with an exotic background that makes her very desirable. Still he is puzzled to see the insolence and abruptness with which she treats her male colleagues. Maybe she does she not know she is a woman.

The barbarian leader suggests that an exchange take place, that he trade the lovely slave girl for the haughty anthropologist. Naturally the men refuse. That night, in the shell of the wrecked ship, in their makeshift camp within it, Dr. High and Mighty heaps scorn on the barbarians, and is much amused at their preposterous suggestion. It is as though they had asked them to trade her, a high-order, highly educated, extremely intelligent human being, one of their own crew members, a person, for an ox or a pig or a camel.

In the morning, however, their camp is surrounded. by hundreds of barbarian soldiers. Clearly they intend to have the woman, if necessary by force. Resistance is useless. The woman is to be theirs, either with or without bloodshed. The men's choice is quite simple. Either they surrender her willingly or, after they are slain, she is taken by force.

"Do not give me up!" she cries, for the first time in her life understanding the dependence of women on the voluntary protection of men. Her Ph.D. forgotten, she finds herself appealing to them as a woman, begging them to defend her.

"Take her," says the leader of the Earth men. "She is yours."

She is is forced to her knees. Chains are snapped on her wrists, slave chains. She is led away, crying and screaming, a weeping, captive, terrified female.

As part of the original bargain, the beautiful alien slave girl remains. She kisses the feet of the men and begs to serve them. The women of this world love men and, as women, wish to be women, the women of such men. They find their pleasure and fulfilment in being women, not in being pseudo-men. There is no hypocrisy and pretence in their loving submission to their masters. They do not dream of the honour of being a free person, or a wife. It is no longer within their nature. They most respond to a man who understands their true nature, and will keep them in their place. They have no respect for a man who pretends not to be dominant. He is like a lion who pretends to enjoy feasting on vegetables, perhaps not even a lion at all, surely, at least, an imposter. Who does he think he is fooling? He is a man, and they are only women. They despise him for his weakness, or his hypocrisy. If they can, they will make his life miserable. They wish to be the doe cornered in his lair. They are pleased most when they lie stripped beneath his paws, held down as his desired prey, feeling his great, rough tongue on their beauty.

The Earth men make their first mistake with the lovely slave when they attempt to treat her with excessive kindness. Sensing this in them as weakness she immediately becomes petty and lazy, irritable and petulant. When the leader, putting aside his scruples, his Earth conditioning, cuffs her twice, bringing blood to her mouth, she realizes, suddenly, that these men, as much as the men of her own planet, are males, and must be obeyed. This brief administration of physical discipline works a transformation in the girl, and, thenceforward, deliciously, joyfully, she serves them. They have demonstrated their dominance over her, and their refusal to accept insubordination. She has tested them, and found them strong. Reassured, knowing now they are truly men, truly her masters, she serves them happily and marvellously as a slave girl. She has forced them to teach her the lesson she desperately wished to be taught. No slave girl wants a weak master. It degrades them. All female slaves desire strong, masculine masters.

After some months, the aliens return again. This time they bring with them a new, beautiful slave girl. She wears scanty, diaphanous garments, rude, barbaric ornaments, sensual, slave cosmetics. She is, of course, Dr. Vivian Stephenson, who has now been trained as a slave girl. Obediently, submissively, as the other slave girl had done, she serves them all food and drink. The Earth men are astounded. They had never realized she was so beautiful. They are further startled at her submissiveness, her unquestioned, self-effacing servility. Through her transparent garments they see that her thigh has been branded. About her throat, however, there is no collar.

The barbarian chieftain, before leaving, again proposes an exchange of women. Vivian looks at the men. pleading with them to accept her. They have, of course, in the past months, grown fond of their young alien slave. Vivian's eyes plead with them. She dares not speak, of course. The men look at one another, and understand one another. The trade is agreed upon. Before departing with his former slave, the barbarian chieftain gives the leader of the Earth men an object, wrapped in silk.

The Earth men, and Vivian, now returned to them, go into the wrecked ship, in which they have their makeshift camp. She is almost hysterically grateful at her rescue. She weeps. She is now safe.

"If you only knew," she weeps, "what they made me do, what they made me learn!" The men, of course, have a very good idea of the training to which the beautiful Earth woman was subjected. She stands there and faces them, clad in the barbaric ornaments of a slave girl.

"Bring me my coveralls," she commands them.

The men do not move.

She is suddenly startled. "Bring me my coveralls!" she demands.

The men regard one another. It is unlikely that they will ever be rescued.

"We do not need now a Ph.D. in anthropology," one of them says to her.

"What do you need?" she asks, in a whisper.

"A woman," responds the leader of the Earth men.

Vivian looks at them, shaking her head. "No," she whispers. "No!"

The leader of the Earth men unwraps the object, wrapped in silk, which had been given to him as a parting gift by the chieftain of the barbarians. It is a steel slave collar.

Vivian looks at him with horror.

"Kneel to be collared, Slave," orders the leader of the Earth men.

Numbly, obediently, Vivian, the female slave, kneels to be collared.

The collar snaps about her throat.

"Whose slave are you?" asks the leader of the Earth men.

Vivian looks about at them. "I am your slave," she whispers, "— Masters."

The leader of the Earth men then takes her in his arms and carries her to a room in the ship, where he places her on his bedding. The others will, in their turn, similarly enjoy the beautiful slave.

This is a rich and complex fantasy, with various roles. In particular, there are two major female roles, those of the anthropologist and the alien slave girl, and two major male roles, those of the leader of the Earth men and the leader of the barbarians. The scientist's roles are relatively easy to perform. A white lab coat is extremely adaptable and combined with a pocket protector and some thick glasses can be very effective. Slave girl costuming is discussed at length in Appendix 3. Barbarian warriors are perhaps the most fun. For inspiration, I suggest the classic Conan tales of Robert E Howard. In the fantasy world of antediluvian Hyboria, Barbarians are tribal warriors, hailing from the the wastelands of the Frozen North, Cimmeria, Pictland, and the Black Coast. While the mercenaries and elite janisseries of Aquilonia,

Nemedia and Stygia are often highly trained professionals, the vast majority of Barbarians are warriors from birth. Their fierce bonds of loyalty are often enough to drive individual barbarians to mighty, near legendary feats of heroism. Leather and pelts are the most favoured items of apparel, although the more accomplished warriors may have acquired a taste for uniforms in their mercenary travels. An extra touch that does well to suggest savagery is the the painted face. This could be the indigo pigments of the Scottish clansmen that fought alongside Braveheart or it could be the black and red stripes that have been more recently popularized by the rock band Turisas. Of course there is also the war paint of indigenous Indians, a style that has been replicated over and over again in contemporary culture.

This entire fantasy, is set in the context of a conflict between two very different cultures. These roles can be played out in sequence. Dr. Stephenson is first at the mercy of the barbarian chieftain, who doubtless teaches her swiftly and well what it is to be a female slave, perhaps even to the kiss of the whip; she is secondly at the mercy of her own crew men, and particularly at that of the leader. The leader of the Earth men, for his part, along with his fellows, learns to his pleasure what it is to be served as a master by the lovely alien slave girl. He is doubtless sexually aroused, and his vanity is pleased, to be the master of a beautiful, helpless female slave, who must serve him intimately and deliciously in all respects. He further learns, of course, that such a wench is most superb and responsive when, to her pleasure, she is subject to the strictest of masculine discipline, when she is most thoroughly and uncompromisingly mastered. Later, of course, the leader of the Earth men, and his fellows, have a new slave girl, a beautiful, exquisite one, the statuesque, enslaved Dr. Stephenson. They will treat her, we may suppose, with vengeance for her former arrogance.

Instructions on How to Purchase a Slave

Slaves are always purchased naked. Only a fool buys a clothed woman. Restrained slaves should always be temporarily freed for ease of inspection and assessment. Private sales, of course, allow more intimate inspection of the merchandise. Have her turn before you, slowly, head back, hands clasped behind her head. If you are alone with the slave and her seller, you have an excellent opportunity for examination, much better than if they are stood on a block, some distance from you, on the block. Order her to walk and move before you, and to lie down, and rise, and kneel, and look over her shoulder, etc. It is possible to tell a great deal from such simple things. Also, stand before her, hold her by the arm, and look down into her eyes. You will then sense the chemistry between you. Look carefully while you grip her. Do her eyes tell you that she fears you, or that you excite her, against her will, or that she will try, desperately, to resist you? Feel her body, her ankles, her calves, the buttocks, her abdomen, her breasts, and her throat. Do you like the feel of her? What is the length and condition of her hair? Open her mouth and examine her teeth. These will tell you a great deal about her general condition. Do not afraid to be rough with her; she is property and she expects it. Examine her candidly; is she young enough to have a good resale value? How many masters has she had? Why did her last master sell her? Was she a bred slave or a capture? If she was bred, what is the reputation of the house that bred her? What sort of training do they give her? If she is a capture, what sort of training, if any, has she received? What is her general background, if of free birth? What, roughly, is her intelligence? Can she cook, iron, clean, wash, sew, etc.? Has she been taught to serve foods and wines? (You might wish to use her as a table slave, as well as a sex slave.) If you are not very wealthy, perhaps you can only afford one girl. You wish to make a sound purchase, and, considering possible resale, a good investment. Test her sexual responsiveness. If the merchant, in a private sale, does not permit this, he is not a bona fide dealer. Lastly, if the merchant is willing (this varies from merchant to merchant), try her out.

If the girl seems, on the whole, acceptable, you may purchase her. Be sure to receive a bill of sale, and her registration papers, suitably endorsed. Little then remains but to lock her in slave cuffs, hood her, put her on a leash, and take her home. At your threshold you unhood her and remove the leash. You leave the cuffs on her; then you throw her to your shoulder and carry her into your home. This is a symbolic act, indicative that she is captive; it is done even though she was purchased. Within moments of entering your house, initiate her to her servitude with the whip. The first thing you do with her inside is to beat her, and then use her. Later she may be set about her work. She must learn from the first instant that you are her master; and that she is complete slave.

Some men prefer to buy from the block; it is very exciting to do so, and the girl, stimulated by the buyers, almost always presents herself well. Some auction sales, maintain exhibition cages with lot numbers, in which the slaves may be observed closely before being bid upon. These exhibits take place on the afternoon of the sale; the actual sale takes place at night; naked women on the block, under torchlight, are very beautiful. Some men, incidentally, like to buy from friends or private owners; sometimes exchanging slaves for a trial period. A purchase from a private owner is sometimes less expensive; the slaver's commission is avoided.

Documentation, Return on Investment and Breeding

It can be great fun to prepare a bill of sale and registration papers on your new slave. Such papers might include biographical data, including capture report, date of branding, processing, training, etc., with appropriate stamps and signatures. Her medical condition, similarly, certified, should appear in these papers, with perhaps a categorization of her sexual responsiveness, for example, is she an "A" female, a "B," or a "C," etc.? (As she learns, these ratings might be updated; if she should become complacent, they might be reduced. A high sex rating is much in a girl's interest, incidentally; it raises her price and tends to assure her a richer master, and a comparatively easier life). These papers should include, too, measurements, for example, height, weight, hips, waist and bust; and, perhaps, left ankle and throat, the former for slave-anklet size, if wished, the latter, of course, for steel-collar size. Some alien cultures might not be interested in measurements that we do not customarily make; for example, what does she measure from the right armpit to the right hip, from the back of the knee to the back of the ankle, etc.; perhaps there are blanks on the forms for these measurements to be entered, and others; in measuring her, of course, treat her roughly; she is only an animal, a slave; the measurements, too, should perhaps not be in inches but in a similar, small unit, on a suitably marked tape, appropriate to another culture. For example, what is her waist size or bust size in Stygian cubits or some other archaic increment? It seems appropriate that slaves, animals, would not be measured as human beings, or high-order rational creatures. They would have their own measures; this distinguishes them from free persons and confirms, in their own mind and that of others, their essential differences from free individuals; a girl, for example, might only know her weight and sizes in slave measures. The sex ratings mentioned previously, as well as other measures and categories, might be similarly "alienized"; this helps the female to think of herself as a slave and gives an exciting "alien reality" to the fantasy; for example, sex ratings in Stygia might not be based on "A's" and "B's," etc., but on a 100-point temperature scale; the sex rating would be a function perhaps of the rapidity with which the slave can be brought to orgasm, combined with the frequency of the orgasms and their intensity; any girl who has a rating of over, say, ninety degrees, might be quite good; she might be the sort of woman who, under a man's touch, in spite of herself, is spontaneously and helplessly responsive. Slavery itself immediately, startlingly, effects a considerable improvement in a female's sexual performance; it is not unusual for a 20-degree free woman, struck and collared, hurled to her master's bed, not permitted inhibitions, to give performances in terror in the seventies and eighties, sometimes in the nineties, sometimes, in unusual cases, in the high nineties.

These papers might also include fingerprints for the purpose of identification; the girl kneels, incidentally, while her prints are taken. In addition, you might also take a print of the large toe of the right foot; this indignity, for some reason, outrages Earth women of free birth. More sophisticated slave identification, and tracking might also be commonplace in more advanced cultures. These might range from sub-dermal bio-chips to a laser beam that inscribes a slave registration number on the bone of the skull, painlessly, through the scalp. These can then be read by suitable scanning devices, The papers will certainly contain pasted-in photos; she might be stripped, kneeling and chained, with pictures front and side view, of her head only.

There should also be endorsements, indicating her changes of ownership, with dates and stamps. The new owner's signature, seller's with stamp, and counter-signature, goes on the last blank line. (This helps to build up the characterization of the female, giving her a "slave history." Perhaps there is a form for reporting the escape of a slave, which is, say, finished off when she is apprehended. What about a form for leasing a slave, or renting her? What about, say, "want lists," submitted to dealers, when you are looking for a given type female. A natural document here, of course, could be a capture order, or slave requisition for reduction to bondage. Perhaps a down payment is made to the slaver, in a sort of contract, the balance to be paid when the wench is delivered, stripped, now nameless, chained and branded, ready for the collar. Finally there is the ownership brand. A red magic marker can be used to make an artistic looking device on a concealed part of the flesh.

One of the main functions of a slave is to entertain. Make your sex slave put on a show. Lean back on your bed and watch as he or she strips, then begins to masturbate for your voyeuristic pleasure. Be sure to issue a command here and there – "slower," "faster," "turn to face me," "spread your legs wider" — or even move them around, repositioning arms or legs to get a better view. In the world of fantasy there are many slave dances. Needless to say, anyone with a training in expressive dance has a head start in these matters. Not all expressive dances need to be the representation of the growth of a bean plant. Far more appropriate to our purposes are dances to the whip, dances in chains, dances of sexual desire, dances of pretended fear and despair, dances of insolence, dances of rebellion, etc. Many dances, end with a physically expressed, wordless, plea for the touch of the master.

An interesting dance is a tether dance, in which she performs on a lead. Dance is an wonderful way for a woman to express her feelings. Similarly, a woman can erotically stimulate herself by dance. It is hard to dance with sexual passion before a man and not become eager for his physical attention.

45. The Slave Farm

Long before the invention of agriculture, wild animals had to be hunted. This was a very dangerous procedure especially with many of the large prehistoric species that have now gone extinct. Aurocs were three times the size of a modern cow and mammoths almost double the size of a normal elephant. We can only imagine the ferocity of a sabre toothed tiger. It is little surprise then that a selection of animals were tamed and domesticated to provide early man with meat and raw materials. For many hundreds of years, men dived in dangerous shark infested waters for pearls. It is only in the last century that pearl farms have been developed. As humans we take it for granted that the breeding and raising of lesser species is quite normal. It is therefore quite rational to expect that long after first contact, superior and technologically advanced would do the same to us. Maybe there are several differing "slave stocks" in the galaxy, of which the human is only one. If this is the case, we might then imagine an enterprising alien race, one with strong mercantile leanings, establishing a series of slave farms. After the initial investment, which might be considerable, both in time and money, a slave crop would be annually yielded. Numerous quality control systems would be introduced to monitor output, not to mention final training procedures.

Specimens might be crated and sent out on approval, while others might visit the farm and survey the stock personally, examining and interviewing them. Prices would be competitive, and the merchandise, if not found satisfactory, may be returned within one local cycle. Slaves are seldom returned; they are anxious to please their masters. The alternative is not worth thinking about. A slave who is twice returned is placed in a special lot, to be disposed of in bulk at unimportant markets, often as chained gang labour in the cramped confines of the dilithium mines, under the shock rods of the spiderlike overseers.

A breeding facility generally consists high, razor-wire fences, coupled with a force field, set to incapacitate, patrolled by occasional air cars. Within the fence are the facilities. The long dormitory sheds, the mating sheds, with their chains and mating pouches, the food troughs, the examination, administration and medical facilities, etc. On a farm such as this, several thousand young females are kept for breeding. Once they reach the age of twenty-five, they are transferred to other facilities to be disposed of on the market. These women are kept as simple breeding stock, to be regularly inseminated by a selected stock of strong, handsome, strong stud males.

Many of the girls at the breeding facility are bred slaves, and have known only the farms. They were among the most beautiful and servile perhaps, bred from the most beautiful and servile before them. But some of the girls at the breeding unit are captures, freshly snared and hooded on Earth, to be brought here as slaves. Our heroine is one such recent arrival. Due to her beauty and femininity, she is consigned to the breeding farms.

Upon arrival, she was herded with hundreds of other naked girls to the feeding troughs, mercilessly kept in line by the electro-whips and snock-rods of the alien overseers. Rather than being chained for insemination in one of the numbered mating stalls, she decide to make a bid for freedom. During the confusion she noted a patrol vehicle parked within the fence perimeter. Lifting her face from the feeding trough, itself a punishable offence, she noted that the driver was engrossed in conversation with a fellow guard and so slowly she edged her way along the trough. Crawling quickly across the floor she managed to slip beneath the vehicle and to rest her body on the bars of its substructure. Escape is such an uncommon occurrence that no one even noticed her disappearance. Even her fellow slaves did not see for fear of lifting their faces from the feeding trough; the whistle has not yet been blown and none of them wish to feel the pain of the electro whips. The slaves, utterly at the mercy of the guards, are eager to please them. Many of them are little more than bred properties, domesticated animals. Some of them have not even been taught to speak. They run panting to the mating stalls, eagerly placing their wrists and ankles in the shackles. Later in the evening the vehicle goes on its patrol, she waits until it touches down beyond the perimeter and slips free.

Beyond the farm are a series of low hills. She keeps low to the ground using stunted brush for cover, Suddenly the search lights of the breeding facility illuminate the fences and the sirens begin to whine. A breeder is missing. Female 221 of herd 16, series 229, camp 14, i.e., specimen 221-16-229-14. This identification code appears on a small metal plate which is punched into her left earlobe. Patrol cars equipped with large search lights can be seen leaving the facility. Packs of howling, eight-legged hunting beasts are released through the main gates, dragging their attendants on long chain leads. She runs desperately through the undergrowth, knowing that she cannot possibly escape her pursuers. She hides in the brush as an air car glides swiftly overhead, its search light a rapid disk, zig-zagging across the ground. She emerges and runs again. The howling grows closer. She is exhausted. Her feet and legs are bleeding. She can run no more. She falls, fearing that the jaws of the beasts will tear her to pieces. She struggles to her feet, stumbles on, and then falls again. Suddenly, about her neck, a rope draws tight. She has been caught and the noose prevents her from crying out. She turns and looks up. It is not an alien. It is a human male. He is rough. He is an outlaw. Long ago he himself escaped from aliens. He has been living in the brush, usually far from the camp.

She looks at him, her eyes wild.

"Greetings, Slave," he says. He speaks in English.

Still, she cannot speak and so he loosens the rope, just slightly.

"I am not a slave," she protests.

His hand lashes out, snapping her head viciously to one side. There is a hot, sticky smear of blood at the side of her mouth. Her lip has been split. She is bleeding. She tastes blood in her mouth.

She feels it on her left breast. She looks at him with horror. She can scarcely comprehend. No man of Earth would have done that.

"Be silent, Slave," says the man.

The rope tightens, choking her, then loosens again.

"Yes," she says.

Yes, what?" he demands.

"Yes—Master," she whispers.

He forces her roughly to the ground with his boot as another air car passes overhead.

Once it has disappeared, he gags her. Then, with his fist hooked into the rope at her throat he drags her to his concealed mount, an oversized kangaroo type beast with shaggy fur and vicious looking tusks. The howling of the hunting beasts grows nearer. Now bound hand and foot she is slung over the bow of the saddle and they make good their escape. She has escaped from one slavery, to that of another, to that of a man.

At first, he sees her as little more than an animal. She is allowed to perform menial, servile tasks. She tries to escape but he quickly recaptures her and from then on she is bound tightly to avoid such a re-occurrence. As punishment he beats her severely with a rude switch. She is left with little choice but to break beneath his will, She finally accepts that she is a slave and he is her master. "I am your slave," she tells him, "please be kind to your slave, Master." No longer does she wish to flee him. She fears now only that she might not sufficiently please him. Gradually, over time, he softens toward her, but still he keeps her always, completely and perfectly, in her place. As she lies in his arms she does not know whether to pity or envy unmastered women; she envies them their freedom but pities them that they have not known a man such as hers.

46. The Tribute

Only a few years into the near future, Earth has been conquered by an alien planet, the population of which is, technologically, far advanced beyond ours. Earthlings, and Earth governments, are terrified. We are completely at the mercy of our alien overlords. If we do not cooperate with them, completely and without any form of resistance, selected cities will be randomly obliterated. Some have been destroyed already, just to prove a point. If necessary, the Earth itself may be destroyed. The aliens do not wish to inhabit the planet Earth. They instead wish to use it primarily as a resource for raw materials. Along with shipments of our most abundant resources, one of the most shocking demands to insure our survival is that each month, one thousand of the most beautiful Earth females must be paid to the aliens as tribute. All Earth women between the ages of sixteen and fifty-five must register, be tabulated and examined. The selection, processing and transportation of the monthly tribute is globally organized and systematic. Our highest levels of computer technology are applied to the selection of optimum tribute. This is a tiny proportion compared to planet's total population. The armed forces, of course, have disbanded and the strongest males are instead drafted to fight as auxiliaries for the aliens in interplanetary wars.

Except for the monthly tributes and shipments, and the fact that the alien flag must be flown, with precedence, with national flags over public buildings, there is not a great deal of difference between the old Earth, free, filled with bickering nations, and the new Earth, a colony planet. Colonisation has been practised in many forms over the centuries and so life goes on much as it normally would. If anything the situation is even better than it was before. Suddenly we have access to incredibly high levels of technology and the world is free from the conflicts that plagued the rest of our history.

Selected women, now receive notifications to report for examination and assessment, for possible inclusion in tribute shipments. They would, in effect, be drafted for such shipments, much as, previously, men were drafted for service in the armed forces. The girls are examined with great care, both medically and psychologically. They are tested and probed in great detail. Only the most beautiful, most healthy, most intelligent, most sexually responsive, are selected. These women do not return. It is not known to what purpose they are applied.

The preceding scenario sets up a situation within which exciting fantasies can be created.

Suppose that your partner, received her "notice." The entire resources of her society are marshalled to see that she reports and, if qualified, takes her place in the tribute quota. Does she attempt to flee? What are her reactions? Was she content with the system, perhaps happy with it, because of the end of war, etc., until she discovered that it might be she herself who would pay this price? Why do the aliens want women? If she tries to flee, do the special police used in such matters catch her and take her, in handcuffs, to the induction and examination station?

The male partner acts a large number of male roles in this fantasy. He may be the policeman who captures her, and forces her to accompany him to the induction and examination station. He may be the examining physician, before whom she must strip herself and be medically assessed. He may be the examining psychologist. Perhaps the police and physicians, etc. are aliens, conducting these matters to their own precise satisfaction? Perhaps the girl is strapped on a special examination table and electrodes are taped to her head and body, their inputs being fed to instruments with gauges and meters. Her erogenous zones are stroked and her responses, with scientific precision, are registered by needles on the gauges and meters. This particular specimen is extremely sexually responsive. She is chosen, perhaps over other women, even more beautiful. How is she fed and restrained before shipment? How is she shipped? Is she drugged and crated? Are there special cells on the space ship that will transport her and others? What is her number? Is her number on a metal plate which is fastened about her neck by a chain or is she branded in a more lasting fashion? What happens to her on the ship? What happens to her when she arrives on the alien world?

Some couples might prefer a historical setting to an interplanetary milieu. In this case it is easy to imagine that the invading Romans have demanded a tribute from the barbarian hordes. The most delectable your females will be shipped off to the capital where they will be enslaved as temple prostitutes. Alternatively the Mongolian conquerors are now demanding that the ordinary Han Chinese select the very best of their eligible females and transport them to the capital where they will serve as imperial concubines.

Of course the conquerors need not always be male. Imagine for a moment a race of fierce Amazonian warrior women. After subjugating the general population in some distant realm, they demand regular tribute of the most attractive male specimens. These unfortunate wretches are rounded up on a regular basis and then bound in servitude as sex slaves to the Wild Women of Wongo.

47. The Unwilling Mind

Imagine that you had no desire to go shopping and yet, suddenly, to your horror, your body got up, put on its hat and coat, left the house and went to the store. However much you fight this with your will, your body, as though in some hypnotic state, performed precisely of its own accord. Anyone watching would never guess that you were possessed by a force not of your own. It even smiles and says "Hello" to people, acting as though nothing unusual were going on. You, however, wild with horror, cannot control its actions. Your will and your mind are a prisoner within your physical being. Your body is now acting autonomously, completely "on its own."

Now imagine for a moment that this autonomy is the result of a new and revolutionary technological development. You are a beautiful woman and you encounter a man to whom you are attracted, but of whom you are also frightened. The handsome stranger is an electronics genius and he points a small device at you which emits an unseen ultrasound signal. Suddenly your body begins to behave toward him as that of a hopelessly enamoured female. You accompany him, helplessly, to his room. You seductively remove your clothing. You dance erotically for him. At his signal, you swiftly leap into his bed, where you lie provocatively, awaiting his caress. You arms are wide open awaiting his embrace, your lips pursed awaiting his kiss. You are fighting from within but you are unable to help yourself. Instead you surprise yourself by making mad passionate love to him. Electronically, against your will, you are forced to engage in the most intimate carnal relations. Your performance is incredible. You even say things to him that shock you. Most amazing of all, you experience the best orgasm of your entire life.

When it is all over, he gets up and prepares to leave. As he exits through the door, he takes out the small electronic object, and turns off its signal, releasing your body to your own control again. You are horrified, naked in bed. You know you cannot charge rape for many saw you come, lovingly and willingly, to the room. As he leaves, he pockets the electronic device and tells you that he will see you again soon.

A interesting variant of this fantasy, which is also powerful, permits the woman to express herself very vocally in speech, while her body, against her will, lovingly performs. "I hate you," she weeps, while performing with great skill and perfection. This fantasy can be an excellent one for a woman who finds sex difficult. Her will can be as much against sex as she pleases. It is her body which must act, whether she willing or not, as that of a passionate woman. This fantasy permits her the luxury of the theoretical rejection of sex coupled with its most detailed and intimate behavioural consummation. She may feel any way she wants, but she must act as though she were a hopelessly enamoured, skilful, passionate lover. In the now well known 'fake it till you make it' technique, a coherence develops between her acting and her feeling. Acting like a hopelessly enamoured, skilful, passionate lover, she might suddenly discover, to her horror, that she is such a woman. Perhaps, at the end, she can resist no longer and, with her full will, her rigidity crumbled, yields herself to him, completely. He looks into her eyes. She is now his, completely. "Yes," she tells him, "I belong to you now. I yield myself to you fully." The electronic device, then, of course, is no longer needed. She is now, truly, his hopelessly enamoured, passionate lover. We may suspect, as well, that her skills, and her wonderfully uninhibited intimacy, originally electronically induced, will not desert her.

Of course, in this age of sexual equality, it is not necessarily only women that might succumb to such a powerful technology. There is no reason why this kind of device could not have been developed by a wealthy Chinese heiress. She has inherited a 'Shanzhai' style fabrication lab in Shenzhen, Wenzhou or maybe even Hong Kong. She now travels the world, forcing men to submit to her will, transforming them into her personal sex slaves. She then has them satisfy her voracious appetite and kinky fetishes, of which she has many. At least this was the scene that I set up with a very special Hong Kong lover a few years ago. There is of course, no reason why you cannot adapt it to fit your own situation and geographical location.

I learned much about this scenario from a friend who is very interested in erotic hypnosis. It is a long-time interest of his and he has over the years developed considerable expertise in the subject. His wife is into it now, too. She she just does not realize it yet.

48. THREESOMES AND AWESOME MORESOMES

The classic ménage à trois is one of the most popular male fantasies of all time. Double your pleasure, double your fun; sex with two lovers is more fun than one! It is a staple of video porn and erotic literature but I can assure that not everything always goes as planned. Before I give you some useful tips for successful threesomes, I would like to retell a few personal tales of how things can quickly turn awkward without proper planning and preparation. Threesome fantasies can be so vivid, especially if one of the partners is your real-life lover, that many people try breathing life into them. The resulting reality spans from having a beautiful experience which enhances your relationship, as well as your sense of your sexual self, to an awful, awkward incident that hurts everyone involved. One thing is for certain: Everything in any fantasy is "perfect" as far as your libido is concerned. Reality, however, is not quite so in tune with what turns you on, let alone what turns on your real-life partner or the third party.

My first few threesome experiences were disastrous. The first occasion that it happened was when I was out partying with two college friends who also happened to be lesbians. When the club closed the three of us jumped into a taxi, and I thought that I would just carry on to my place once I had dropped them of at theirs. As it happened they offered me their sofa while we were in the cab, so I jumped out with them and went inside. We went into the kitchen to get some food and the next thing I know, the hole in one's tights was being played with by the other girl. The hole eventually gets big enough for her to put her hand in, and as it is right next to her crotch, she ended up fingering her girlfriend. I got a raging hard-on pretty damn quick. Next thing I know there is a hand on my fly and shortly after that everyone's clothes were off.

I am sad to say that it was the worst experience of my sex life so far. The two girls proceeded to pleasure each other, with my fingers and tongue just getting in the way. I was absolutely forbidden to put my dick near either of them. I ended up jacking off on the edge of their bed as a total spectator. When they had satisfied each other and gone to sleep, I got up, put on my clothes and walked back to the main road to flag down a cab.

Disheartened but not completely put off, I decided to try again when the opportunity next offered itself. This time I went home with two Asian party girls. They were hot but unwilling to get sexual with each other. Turned into an awkward physical workout on my part. Having two women at the same time is surprisingly difficult. In some ways, it is like trying to perform two completely different actions with either hand at the same time, but only with your entire body. A bit like patting your head and rubbing your tummy, except with your dick and two girls. I later leaned that the secret was to pat with your dominant hand and begin rubbing before you start patting, although it was not much help on the threesome front. When one was sitting on my lower body and the other on my face, I would find myself focusing more on the humping than on the licking - so I would be happily humping away while my tongue was just sort of hanging out of my mouth doing nothing. Noticing this, I would suddenly focus more on the tongue and then my lower half would lapse into a sort of half-hearted hump. Like I said, it was difficult. We had fun, but it was difficult. Ideally, in a FMF threesome the two girls she be into each other, or if not into each other at least both into you. Otherwise you have a series of twosomes with a spectator who you know is impatiently waiting for their turn... and a LOT of condom switching.

I have a friend that has been in a polyamorous relationship with two women for over five years. They all live together and the two women are both bisexual. They have threesomes all the time. The three of them are very liberated and a little bit freaky too. Sad thing was that as a guy he would finish two or three times in a night and then he is done. Not so with them of course, they can go for hours and hours. Usually after about an hour he goes to play Xbox while they wear themselves out. It just goes to show that if you get enough of something it becomes old hat, no matter how amazing it might seem. He maintains that two women sleeping in his bed all the time is nothing short of awesome. Having two women to help out around the house, to share the bills, to keep him company when he is lonely are just a few of the advantages. On the other hand there are two women to fight with when things go bad. Having to make up to two after the fight? Not awesome. Not getting as much alone time as he wants? And when the two women have issues between themselves and he is trying to keep them both happy? Definitely not so awesome. Like any other relationship, there are really great things and really bad things. The only thing is it can be a lot more complicated and exhausting at times. He does consider himself lucky but it is not the 24/7 blistering hot fuck-fest that most people imagine. He describes it as "living every man's dream and nightmare at the same time." Relationships are always hard between two people; three is going to be exponentially more difficult.

Still, it is preferable to the experience of another friend who found himself in a threesome fantasy. Once he was spent they simply kept going without him. He was sat in a chair catching his breath when he heard his girlfriend make a noise that he had never heard from her before. Needless to say she left him shortly after for her new friend.

Ever experimental, I decided to try a devil's threesome instead. This involves two males and one female. This was at a lady friend's request and went reasonably well apart from one instance where she was on all fours servicing both of us at each end. I was getting blown while my male friend was doing her from behind. Eventually he got carried away and every time he thrust I got head-butted in the pubic bone, while she made a weird choke/grunt sound. I began hearing a muffled BAAAA in my mind and it was very much like getting a blow job from an irritable mountain goat.

The MMF combination initially seems like it has the potential to be a less awkward situation but that is not always the case, especially if the two dudes decide to spaz out if they cross swords. I heard about one devil's three-way from a friend that ended with the words,

"If your balls touch my knee one more time dude, I'm gonna punch your dick off."

"Excuse me? If your knee touches my balls one more time this is going up your ass, not hers."

This underlying tension might stem from the fact that our society is more homophobic than lesbian-phobic. Modern ladies also seem to have an easier time accepting their bi-curious fantasies than most men do. Masters and Johnson reported that heterosexuals often fantasize about homosexual encounters and vice versa, more often reflecting curiosity and other impulses than the desire to change the gender of one's real-life lovers. Our society tends to make things black or white, good or bad, male or female, heterosexual or homosexual. But the human sexual imagination is most definitely bisexual, even what you might call omnisexual. Men are not from Mars, and women are not from Venus. We are all from the same beautiful, wild, sexual planet Earth, and we are far more alike than we are different. Human sexuality exists on a vast and beautiful spectrum. Dr. Alfred Kinsey was among the first to show that we are all on a bisexual continuum with absolute heterosexuals on one end and absolute homosexuals on the other end. Very few of us fall at one extreme or the other. Most of us are bisexual to some degree. That does not mean we like both sexes equally at all times. It just means that most of us can potentially, under the right circumstances (boarding school, prison, the armed forces, etc.), with the right person (the perfect lover), be aroused by either gender.

Fortunately, I have since had a number of much more positive threesome experiences and can happily recommend the activity to anybody. One particular girlfriend was especially kinky and wanted to be double teamed by me and another girl in a three way incest fantasy. I played the role of Papa, the second girl was Mama while she age-played as our little daughter.

One evening, I was approached by a woman at a bar and chatted with her and her brother for an hour or so. He ended up leaving us and we decided to go back to her place to hang out. We ended up having some really wild sex but as I rolled off her to use the bathroom I noticed her "brother" standing in the doorway, fully naked, with his cock in his hand. Turns out he was actually her husband and he enjoyed watching her with other men.

After the initial shock wore off they asked me to help with a fantasy that they had. They wanted to do the same thing the next night but have me break in and pretend to rape her only to have him come home, put a gun to my head and sodomize me while I was still inside of her. Maybe the biggest sexual WTF moment of my life and definitely the fastest NO of my life.

The only way to successfully have a threesome is to both agree beforehand to focus on the third partner. Otherwise it is uneven and there will always be negative feelings. Instead of pleasuring each other, put all your energy to the third person. Use them as a conduit to share this experience. Gang up on them if you have to. If you do not, there is going to be an awkward sense of jealousy. If the two of you are already a couple and are meeting a third party, then one person should actively take charge. Be immediately physical with hugs and kisses, which will help to break the ice. If you are very detail-oriented, threesomes can become confusing. You quickly lose track of who is at which stage and there is lots of ambiguous moaning. Ideally, everybody should be trying to divide their attention equitably so that that there is no clear twosome or onesome.

Threesomes are of course not for everybody. Some people are petrified even at the thought of having to share their partner in a three way situation. If you do not even feel comfortable with your dog being in the bedroom while you are fooling around then this is a pretty good signifier that threesomes may not be for you. If on the other hand you want to start slowly, then try acting out a threesome fantasy using sex toys first. A vibrator can take the place of an additional partner and make it easier to gauge your partner's reactions to the whole concept. As a next step you could always try visiting a strip club together. If you both like watching each other enjoying lap dances, then it might be time to discuss taking this fantasy to the next level.

One interesting twist on the MFM threesome is as follows. If your girlfriend shows interest in this and you can find a friend to help out then then try this. Have her wear her sexiest (read sluttiest outfit) outfit, perhaps a mini skirt and fishnets. Blindfold her and tell her that you have arranged to fulfil her fantasy. In our case, I had her pleasure me orally, so that I could grab her head as my friend made his entrance and prevent her from moving. The mystery man never spoke. Instead I verbalized plenty of filthy talk to keep her excited. Once we had ravaged her to her heart's desire my friend got up to leave. The really delicious part was that I never told her who it was and she could never look the same way at any our friends again, partly out of embarrassment and partly out lust.

A threesome can easily become an orgy, which is another common sexual fantasy. One way to keep sexual monogamy from becoming monotony is to maintain an active fantasy life with as many different partners as you can imagine. Unfortunately as the number of participants increases so does the potential for problems. Gang-bangs in particular are extremely difficult to arrange, and you will have to worry about keeping your girl safe if someone tries to get out of hand. Also bear in mind that this kind of behaviour does not go down well in certain locations. Despite its vast prostitution industry, orgies remain a criminal offence in China. Ma Yaohai, a 53-year-old college professor and 21 other members of a swingers' club in the Chinese city of Nanjing, were recently jailed for the crime of "group licentiousness." Ma was jailed for three and a half years while eighteen others ranging including ordinary white-collar workers, taxi drivers and sales clerks were sentenced for up to two and half years. "Ma received a more severe punishment because he did not admit the malicious and illegal nature of his conduct," the court in eastern Nanjing said. The largest online site about group sex, Happy Village, has more than 380,000 registered members. Extramarital affairs and prostitution are commonplace all over China and many corrupt officials secretly have multiple mistresses. Even so, because such activities are often restricted to the wealthy and to government officials, they are in practical terms exempt from prosecution. China regularly uses the so-called charge of "hooliganism," a catch-all term that criminalized everything from premarital sex to dancing with members of the other sex and listening to Western music. During the early 1980s, a woman was sentenced to death for participating in secret dance parties.

If you are in a country where the general attitude is liberal and free then there are a number of ways to get an orgy started. One of the easiest is to arrange a session of strip poker or the like. This experience can be enhanced with the following suggestions:

Everyone at the gathering will be told in advance exactly how many articles of clothing to wear. Therefore, there will be no advantage for the "cold" person in the room.

Alcohol does "lubricate" the situation. The warm-up hands should be played with Jello shots in extra small cubes.

All bets are "one" or "double." So at the most, you bet one or two articles of clothing at a time. There are no blinds or antes.

Once all clothing is removed for someone, out comes two bowls and a digital timer. One bowl contains "dare" and the other one contains "double dares." So instead of articles of clothing, you are betting dares or double dares (one or two). Dares are relatively easy stuff (go sit on someone's lap and kiss them for ten seconds, go lick their nipple for ten seconds, get your penis hard) while the double dares are a bit more daring (perform oral sex on someone for 15 seconds, kiss everyone in the room's genitals, etc.)

If after a short time, the game has not been forgotten and the sex is not rolling, make it more explicit with a triple dare bowl which can include acts of penetration. Strip Yahtzee and strip Monopoly usually take a little longer but can achieve the same ends.

49. The Virgin Sacrifice

As most people already know, sex with a virgin can be extremely overrated. This is because the true sexual connoisseur understands that the real excitement comes not from deflowering virgins but sacrificing them to demanding pagan gods.

The process is quite simple

Step 1: Acquire virgin.

Step 2: Locate volcano.

Step 3: Full blood orgy with animals

On second thoughts step two might be a little difficult and step three could be off-putting for vegetarian readers so let us look at a completely different approach.

The virginity as an offering the Old Gods fantasy is an enactment filled with exotic detail. In this scenario a beautiful virgin is kidnapped and stripped naked by the celebrants of a strange ancient rite. She is chained, limbs apart, on a cold stone altar as the centre of the ceremony. The chants of the adherents provide a hypnotising soundtrack, their evil guru leading the heretic congregation and the frenzied responses of the faithful. She looks up. A great stone statue, carved with the most triumphal giant phallus looks down upon her helpless, spread-eagled body. In the torch-lit background are statues of other highly sexualised deities of this strange pagan pantheon. Chanting and thick incense fills the air as the worshippers build themselves up into a frenzy of sexual passion. Gradually the pagan priests, by caressing her, arouse her to sexual paroxysm on the altar. She writhes helplessly in her chains. At the wild climax of the ceremony, one of the pagan priests, either himself or with an instrument, deflowers her.

Women tend to fantasize this sort of thing rather well. It is, in fact, a feminine fantasy that will strike a responsive chord in many women. Any fantasy that a woman, intuitively and immediately, can feel in her blood is likely to be capable of delicious enactment for her. For some women it might provide an attractive entry into imaginative sex. Based on the pleasure found in this fantasy she might be encouraged to experiment with many others, gradually building up a repertoire of fantasies, which would produce for both herself and her partner multiple, diverse and incredible dimensions of pleasure.

If the celebrant who ceremonially deflowers her uses an instrument of ceremonial defloration, he must be careful, of course, not to injure her. A finger, used repeatedly, will generally serve the purpose. In many parts of the world, there are now so many sex shops that locating an evil-looking black dildo should be relatively easy. In this context, it is important to remember that the woman receive great pleasure, and not be injured or made uncomfortable.

For practical purposes, the stone alter might be replaced with a dining room table or some other piece of furniture that is raised off the ground. A bed is too comfortable for this purpose. Scented candles and joss sticks are perfectly acceptable substitutes to swinging censers, giant thuribles and incense burners. I personally prefer incense cones to candles. Not only are they less of a fire hazard but cheap Chinese-made candles tend to use synthetic extracts that are extremely overpowering. I will never forget one evening when a female partner reacted very badly to the candles that I had set up and spent most of the evening throwing up in the bathroom rather than orgasming endlessly in the bedroom as I had planned. If you do use candles, make sure that there is plenty of ventilation.

Search carefully online for interesting soundtracks for this fantasy. I like the repetitive sounds of Philip Glass and would recommend parts of Koyaanisqatsi as a suitable aural backdrop. There is also plenty of chanting in the movie Baraka that would also be great in this situation. Perhaps the Afro-beats of Fela Kuti would be useful if you wanted to give the event a voodoo slant. Download the music sharing software known as Soulseek to sample a wide range of ceremonial music from all over the world and then select something that you feel is appropriate.

Chaining a victim can be expensive and time consuming and so

I usually just bind her hands and feet. Silk scarves are my favourite choice but neck-ties are fine too. Previously I have purchased thick curtain cords for this purpose and they too have worked well. If you blindfold the victim for the initial part of the ceremony then it really does not matter what ties you decide to employ.

After the girl's virginity has been publicly sacrificed to the stone god, she is removed from the altar. She is now little more than a simple captive, and is no longer of any religious interest. It would be unimaginative, and a waste of girl, of course, now to simply kill her and dispose of the body. Instead, she is chained to the temple wall, with other girls who had preceded her on similar occasions, as a temple prostitute. The wall is long and low, and a great many girls, naked, are chained to it by the left ankle. They are there for the use of the faithful. They may be sexually enjoyed for the price of a small offering, a small coin, placed in a brass bowl near them, to the god of phallic triumph. This is where the male partner has the opportunity to fulfil his own passions. The girl is already aroused. She is ready for love, and eager for it. She has at least two more orgasms to go. Let us hope he has not forgotten a coin.

50. WIZARDS AND WITCHES

Deemed separate from demonologists and Satanists, wizards are experiencing somewhat of a renaissance in western society. Wicca is the world's fastest growing religion, and thanks to the adventures of Harry Potter, magic of all varieties is enjoying a serious comeback. If you want to make your partner moan like Myrtle or encourage your boyfriend to Slytherin to your chamber of secrets, then this is a rich vein for sexual roleplay. So many women already have fantasies about characters from Lord of the Rings. In fact some might argue that a girl only becomes a woman the day she moves from crushing on Legolas to lusting after Aragorn.

A reliable sign of the popularity of this type of fantasy roleplay is the growing number of vibrators related to this niche genre. Necronomicox are a range of terrifying dildos inspired by the R'lyehian horrors from beyond sanity, of H.P. Lovecraft's Cthulhu stories. Thanks to the rise of 3D printing there is also the the Bad Dragon, an imaginary dragon dick that comes with a full story and truly terrifying fan art. "Fantasy" of this nature no longer simply means "tall dark stranger,"

While the traditional 'hubble, bubble, toil and trouble' crones might not be everybody's idea of hot fantasy, there are plenty of roles to be played out in this genre. My favourite of these is the houri, or nymph of paradise. Born in a seedy part of any medieval city, she grew up poor and miserable but dreamed of a better future. Rather than turning to a life of thievery or prostitution, her beauty and intelligence leads her to a life a magic. Once there, she specializes in charming, enchanting, and seducing. Some look down on her as a common whore and a vixen while others view her as a sensual beauty and the most desirable being on the Prime Material Plane. In addition to magical abilities, houris have a voluptuously alluring beauty and mesmerising charm. She eschews the shapeless robes of ordinary witches, preferring translucent silks and the arresting outfits of oriental concubines. Occasionally she might appear in the conical hat, sexy mini dress and fishnets of a modern Halloween witch. In addition, she has at her disposal a spell book full of magic to invigorate her lovers and incapacitate her enemies. Examples of these invocations include the following

Mordenkainen's Lubrication
Fyltar's Pheromonal Force
Kiss Of Weakness
Phantasmal Lover
Layla's Kiss of Insanity
Stanza's Certain Enchanted Kiss
Conjure Succubus/Incubus
Layla's Seductive Shape-change
Summon Cissaldan
Annihilator's Penis of Power!
Don Juan's Irresistible Kiss

Lipsticks Of The Houri - Sleeping - Wounding - Weakness - Slavery
Periapt Of Sexual Aides
Musk Of Attraction
Philtre of Love
Phylactery of Prophylactics
Potion of Aphrodisia
Potion of Potency
Ring Of The Bulls
Wand Of Love

Their spell casting abilities are clearly rated to sex and seduction. They can charm and fascinate. They possess silver tongues that can influence even the strongest wills. Their love spells are legendary. They are able to enchant and their kiss can cause, confusion, paralysis, and even death.

Houri temptresses are often found in the service of the Temple of Halea or as unusually talented members of the Courtesans' Guild. Such a woman could rise to a position of very great power indeed, perhaps as the wife or mistress of a mighty nobleman or even a King. Houri are considerably more common in the fantasy worlds Robert E. Howard's Conan series. In the realm of Hyboria, they are found in great numbers in the harems of rich Easterners and the Temples of those Goddesses of a more sensual nature, such as Ishtar, the Ivory Goddess, and even those of the Snake-God, Set.

There are even influential historical figures such as Cleopatra and period fiction characters like Milday Duwinter that would certainly qualify as Houri. They have already been embracer by the role-playing gamers with the Sisters of Rapture and the infamous Book of Erotic Fantasy. From Mongoose Publications, we now also have Nymphology and The Quintessential Temptress.

While it is the the Arabic and Islamic myths with a distinct "Sword and Sorcery" flavour that have created the iconic houri, modern myths have embraced the same values. The "femme fatale" character appears in many contemporary works, from Louise Brooks' 'Looking for Lulu' in the silent era all the way up to the Bond girls of modern spy fiction. Who has not heard of the now legendary Mata Hari or the female ninjas from Samurai Japan where they performed the deadly dual role of houri/assassin. Even Star Trek has given us the Deltans and Betazoids, each with strong sexual themes to their cultures. Characters such as Annora and Saffron from the Firefly TV series display an exquisite ability to manipulate or distract both men and women.

APPENDIX 1 - TIES AND BINDINGS

There are literally hundreds of ways to tie a slave. Any man who senses the sexuality of the bound, naked woman is responding to the heritage of the hunter and captor. A woman's body can be especially stimulating to a male in certain contexts, attitudes and postures. Experimentation and mutual discussion are helpful when deciding on ties. Both partners will probably have ideas of certain ways in which they might be bound which would be felt as being "sexy." Find out about these things. Their ideas will be illuminating and you should take advantage of their ingenuity. Imagination and experimentation are both highly desirable characteristics in any sexual partner.

I personally prefer silken cords, strips of cloth and neck ties to rope. Rope does not hold as well, and, if rough rope, may scratch or irritate the skin. One must be careful with bonds. A captive may be perfectly held without being tied particularly tightly. The bonds should be sufficiently tight that the captive knows they are helpless, but they should not be tight enough to pinch or mark the wrists, or slow the circulation. If they beg, in play, that they be loosened, or removed, that may be a cue that they should be tightened, scornfully and callously. One thing to be particularly careful of is any fastening used on the throat. These must always be loose enough to insure free breathing and the individual must never be so situated that they might fall or roll in such a way as to inadvertently tighten such a fastening. Bungee cords make interesting bondage gear. The kind you can find in a hardware store for securing loads to a car are also excellent for restraining. Pad or cover the place where the hooks meet the cord, and latch the cords around the bed. Bungee cords are deceptive; a person bound this way may feel like he or she can escape, but they are surprisingly secure. Cling film or Saran wrap is a fun, sexy bondage implement. Your partner stands with his or her arms at their sides while you wrap them from head to foot in a cocoon. This is a quick, easy bondage technique that is highly secure, and a nude person wrapped in see-through wrap is quite sexy. You can spank, poke, pinch, and otherwise play with any part of your partner's body without any ropes getting in your way; this is very effective when combined with a blindfold. A person wrapped in Saran wrap can easily overheat; it is important to take steps to keep that person cool. A fan works well for this. Also, once the Saran wrap is removed, the person will tend to cool down very quickly; a warm robe is good to have handy.

Some people prefer to be bound in a very specific way. Often times this means above the head to create a feeling of helplessness. Some people will strap their lovers down using a mattress strap that forces their hands down at either side but this can be unsatisfying for some individuals. Tie a strap to your bed frame and run it up the head of your mattress. If you do not have a headboard then consider buying a cheap one on Craigslist and drill in some eye bolts. This way her wrists will move against one another, reinforcing the sense of capture. Her hands are held so far from the body that they are helpless to protect. Make sure that the palms face upward, rather than down toward the bed.

Others are sexually stimulated by having their legs split and having their ankles tied apart to the bedposts. It makes them feel deliciously vulnerable and helpless. Their hands might then be tied, similarly, apart, so that they are completely spread-eagled on the bed.

A simple chained ankle with about five feet of chain, fastened to the leg of the bed is surprisingly effective. Put a comforter on the floor but maintain that this is their place. They can also be chained by the throat or the wrist. Another lead type combination has the hands bound behind the back, with a long length of cord looped several times about the midriff and knotted at the navel. A stick, drilled or notched, is thrust behind her back, and her arms are brought forward under the stick. Her wrists are then lifted and tied, the cords against her belly. Her arms, near the elbows, are fastened to the stick. This keeps the hands tight to the body.

Chains and padlocks suggest slavery more than any rope. A chain which is fastened about the neck and dangles to the floor, to which other chains, for hands and ankles are attached, is very symbolic. Ankle stocks, or wrist stocks, with two openings, are not difficult to make. A simple metal and wood stock can be made by finding a board and two large "U" bolts. The board is drilled. The captive's wrists or ankles are then placed against the board, the "U" bolts inserted over the wrists or ankles, pushed through the board, and, on the other side, behind the board, secured.

The slave hobble is effected by chaining a slave's right wrist to her left ankle, with about a foot of chain. This is particularly effective in that it permits some movement and some resistance, but, frustratingly, teasingly, never enough to be effective.

In a circle tie the wrists are tied behind the back and bound to the ankles, which are pulled back and fastened in proximity to the wrists. This is primarily a holding tie and a captive, thus secured, cannot rise to their feet. This allows them to be fastened about a tree or a post.

A tied sack may be dragged along the floor; it may be lifted in the arms; it may be, under no circumstances, be dropped on the floor; it may, however, be thrown on a bed. A rug may also be used, tied at the four coners. A variation, of course, would be to shut her in a trunk, padlocking it shut. Holes should be drilled, for adequate ventilation. It may also be pretended that under the bed is a low-ceilinged, flat slave cell. With hands bound and ankles crossed and bound, try attaching the slave to the lower bed post. They should be fastened two feet above the floor level. She, thus, cannot rise to her feet. She must lie on her back, under your scrutiny, when you care to look upon her. This tie makes a girl feel helpless. It is always desirable if her head is lower than her feet; this induces a feeling of helplessness and makes the beating seem more painful.

A cangue (also known as a Chinese pillory) is a device that was used for public humiliation and corporal punishment in China, until the early years of the twentieth century. Often the cangue was large enough that the prisoner required assistance to eat or drink, as his hands could not reach his own mouth. It was similar to the pillory used for punishment in the West, except that the board of the cangue was not fixed to a base, and had to be carried around by the prisoner. Although there are many different forms, a typical cangue would consist of a large, heavy flat board with a hole in the centre large enough for a person's neck. The board consisted of two pieces. These pieces were closed around a prisoner's neck, and then fastened shut along the edges by locks or hinges. There was also a label usually listing the offender's name, address, and nature of the crime. The size and especially the weight were varied as a measure of severity of the punishment.

It is always useful to have some kind of linen trunk at the end of the bed. Choose one that locks to hide X-rated toys that do not blend well. Look for one with ring handles to tie your lover down, turn it into a spanking bench, or use it as an impromptu wedge to explore different angles. It might even be trunk sized for crating and shipping captives. If not then consider a collapsible cage and slide it under the beg when not in use.

If your place has support beams, screw a heavy grade hook into the ceiling. When it is not displaying a hanging flower basket or decorative indoor mobile, it can hold a sex swing or provide the catch for a tether that pulls your lover's cuffed hands above his/her head, deliciously naked and vulnerable (without cutting off circulation, of course). Do not suspend loved ones off their feet without advanced training/study of BDSM rope suspension techniques; you can cause serious harm to shoulder joints and tissue.

For beginners, have the slave kneel, head to the floor, ankles under thighs. Her neck is tied to her ankles; her wrists are then bound behind her back. This holds her head to the floor, in a beautiful submission posture. Also her whole body, with its delicious curvatures, is "packaged neatly," confined into a lovely, vulnerable area. This is useful in slave discipline. Slaves are usually whipped on the back (the legs, calves and back of the neck may be included), the stomach or the soles of the feet. Broad, soft leather straps are used, that her back not be cut to pieces, that she be only punished, and not marked. If you are lucky enough to have a harem, try having the punishment administered by one slave girl to another; they hate one another and enjoy striking one another; pettiness, jealousy, mutual distrust, etc., is encouraged in slave girls; it makes them easier to control; the master, after having given his orders, leaves the room; he does not even watch. This is a further insult to the punished girl.

The very first set of ropes that I purchased were cheap, "buy it by the yard" curtain tiebacks. If you are buying ten metres, you might get an odd look from the fabric-store owner but is super soft and very functional. I also like satin ribbons, the kind that are used to wrap wedding presents. The effectiveness of nylon rope depends on the knots and how it is employed in BDSM practice. It is used frequently because it is easy to tie and untie, waterproof (so the knots do not tighten and does not mold easily or retain germs, etc.) and it is more comfortable against the skin. Thickness, braid, etc. can all make a difference as well. Any type of suspension work should proceed with careful study and/or mentorship because it requires skill and expertise to do it the right way. It can cause serious rope burn and it can slip if you are doing partial suspensions.

Small ratchet straps make fantastic tie downs and they make very exciting sounds. A shoulder strap from a duffel bag: makes a great behind the neck leg spreader thanks to the the neck pad. Quick release snaps are available from home improvement shops. These are something thing that you will really need if you are doing any sort of bondage that is more than tying someone down to a bed. These snaps can be released while bearing weight which can be important if your sub/bottom faints in bondage and you need to get him/her down quickly.

Did you know that "Shock Wave" and "Rip Cord" devices were designed for the sole purpose of keeping your surfboard attached to either an arm or a leg, without causing harm to that particular appendage, even in the violent thrashing of a really good wave. Imagine the research that went into the development of this product. Now imagine using these devices for bondage as well-padded wrist and/or ankle restraints, attached to a 6-10 ft piece of 5/16in shock cord.

Parachute cording is both incredibly strong and incredibly soft because its made of pure silk. It can be found in fabric warehouses or military surplus stores. Take a length of rope, at least 3' long. 6" in, make a 180 degree bend and set it so that the bend is between the thumb and index finger of the sub and the loose and long ends of the rope are over their wrist. Take the long end of the rope, wrap once around the loose end and then wrap around the wrist (so that loose end is included) two to three times above the turn around the loose end; then wrap back one to three times below the turn around the loose end. Feed the loose end through the loop and pull. For extra security, tie the remainder of the long end around the loose end. Then, tie the loose end to any anchor or lead. Repeat as desired around other joints (opposite wrist, the ankles, the knees, etc. - but never the neck); and, as with any other type of cuff, do not make it so tight as to cut off circulation.

To make spreader bars, buy the kind of wooden spindles that are used on porch railings. They come in 3ft lengths and vary on width. They come in many shapes, and are ready to paint or stain. Drill the ends and add screw in eye bolts for attaching chains, tethers etc.

Imaginary bondage and mind-control ties involve no physical restraint whatsoever. The captive is merely instructed to place their limbs in certain positions, such as crossing their hands behind their back. Only then do they discover, to their horror, that they cannot move them at all. Their bind is controlled, confined by their own helpless will. Fantasy electronic control devices, including pain collars and implants in neural pain centres are interesting additions to futuristic, technologically-advanced fantasies. I also enjoy the use of magnetic shackle ties. It is supposed that captives wear, on their wrists and ankles, some form of metal rings, perhaps with facing flat plates. They can normally move freely. At a signal, however, from an instrument, these devices snap together, confining them. This permits immediate immobilization of a slave population.

The Knotty Boys first began teaching interactive rope bondage workshops in 1999 at a dungeon venue in San Francisco called

Castlebar. Their goal was to demystify rope bondage, to provide instruction for safe, functional and aesthetically pleasing ties for the bedroom or beyond. They have published two books, Two Knotty Boys: Showing You the Ropes (2006) and Two Knotty Boys: Back on the Ropes (2012). Best of all, on their website they have created over a hundred video tutorials, all available for free download. This is a wonderful resource for beginners and advanced students alike.

http://www.knottyboys.com/code/galleries.php

Appendix 2 - Advanced Bondage and Discipline

Master/slave fantasies are much more common than you might realise. They have some of the most serious erotic charge imaginable. It can be fun to be a sex slave for one night only but if you wish to learn more about this exciting experience then here is a advanced class for newly arrived doms and subs.

Did you know that Angelina Jolie has a love for bondage and previously wore a vial of ex-husband Billy Bob Thornton's blood around her neck? Jolie claimed her experiences with S&M improved her physically, personally, and spiritually. However, these interviews took place in the years prior to her marriage to Hollywood superstar Brad Pitt. Since then, Jolie has admitted that her marriage and family life have taken up the time that she used to commit to whips and chains.

Keep a few things handy. If you want to tie somebody up then have some blunt-nosed scissors on hand in case you need to get them loose in a hurry. Bandage scissors can be slipped beneath a rope without risk of cutting the skin. Handcuffs are flashy and fun, but have to be watched as they can dig into the nerves and do long term damage - only use them if you are not going to be putting a lot of pressure on them. Scarves, pantyhose and ties work well, but do not tie the knots too close to the skin. The point here is to create the aura; later, if you want to follow this path, you can learn how to restrain someone so that they really cannot get away, and do it safely. Stay away from the neck. Never leave your partner bound and unattended with no way to get free. Try binding wrists with a rope of paper towel. Knowing that it is breakable is reassuring for first-timers.

Many men prefer submissive roles due to the fact that it is a change of pace and allows them to be what they are not expected to be. Take complete control, and use phrases like "You know better than that."

Whisper in your lover's ear that "You are now completely under my command." Then proceed to tease them mercilessly until they are literally begging for more. The most important thing to remember is communication. In situations like this, talking about what you like and dislike is very important. You do not necessarily have to tell him or her exactly what you are planning; sometimes surprises are fun. But you do not want to do anything your partner hates, either. Pay attention! Use common sense. Do not rush full-tilt into things you have not tried yet.

Unfortunately a lot of guys are trying to push the boundaries of 'The most epic sexual experience EVAR' and that can lead to some really messed up exotification and 'authentic pleasure' experiences in men. My advice is too keep it simple and relatively vanilla at first. Nobody wants to end up being found hanging in a closet with a belt around their neck and their dick in their hand, dressed in a batman costume. It is not like you need to go for a full lifestyle change and start reading The BDSM Daily and dropping gallons of cash on a rare dungeon furniture imported from Lithuania. You just want something that gets you both going and that saves on lube.

The most effective starting position is kneeling with the hands placed on the thighs. Start with commanding the slave to turn their palms upward. The palm is a very sesitive and sexy area. Trace a design in the palm with a fingernail. Some think that the palm subconsciously represents other more intimate vulnerable parts of the body. Different designs can have different meanings, creating an imaginative method of giving a slave commands.

Tactile senses are enhanced when other senses are taken away. Some BDSM shops make special hoods called "ball hoods" which are designed to cover the eyes and ears but these are expensive and unnecessary, Start instead with a simple sleeping mask. This makes the blindfolded partner feel much more at their lover's mercy. Hoods can also be used, but care must be taken that there is no difficulty or impairment in breathing. A hood, tied under her chin, covering the entire head, can make a slave feel very helpless, particularly if naked.

Direct her by voice command. Since she cannot see, this will be even more frightening to her. Care must be taken, of course, to see that she does not fall. Stay close to her, or be sure to stay between her and any possible danger, such as, say, a coffee table. When she is where you want her tell her to kneel. A blindfold and ear muffs can also work well. For a more high-tech approach, you can use a pair of headphones - the kind that fit entirely over the ear - connected to something that produces static, like a TV with no signal (or even a tape recording of static). In any event, a partner who cannot see or hear will tend to feel other things much more intensely, so combining bondage and sensory deprivation with other ideas works very well.

You do not need to spend a fortune on equipment. Here are a few fun things you can do with everyday objects:

Clothes pegs make wonderful toys as do bag clips. Craft shops will have pegs or clothes-pins in a wide variety of different sizes. They can be clamped to all sorts of interesting parts of the body, and the sensation is quite intense indeed. Furthermore, the longer they stay on, the more intense the sensation when they come off. Clamp them to nipples, or anywhere along the breasts; along the sides, arms, legs, and thighs; and in fact almost any other place you can think of. Generally speaking, plastic clothes pegs produce a more intense sensation than wooden clothes pegs, and smaller pegs have a sharper "bite" than larger ones. A zip strip is made up of six wooden pegs each with a small hole drilled in one handle. Tie the clothes-pins along a piece of cord, leaving about four inches or so between clothes-pins. The result can be clamped in a row along a partner's body. Once the pegs are in place, it is just a matter of finding exactly the right time to tug sharply on the cord, pulling the row of pegs free, one after the other. If you are feeling particularly wicked, tie one end of a long piece of cord to a peg, run it through a pulley in the ceiling, and attach a weight to the other end. Clamp the peg on your partner's nipple or some other suitably erogenous area and have them hold the cord in their teeth. If they let go, the weight will fall and pull the peg off. Now, see what you can do to make them open their mouth.

A pair of chopsticks and a couple of rubber bands can also be used to make improvised clamps. Put the chopsticks above and below nipples, or along each slide of the clitoris, and rubber-band them together at the ends. A clothes hanger with two pincers are perfectly designed as a set of dual nipple clamps.

Spanking toys are available inexpensively from a large range of sources. Wooden spoons are very 'stingy.' Rubber ice scrapers are more of a dull 'thud.'

Cupping sets are popular in Asia but snake bite kits are available inexpensively from camping supply places and department stores. Both include suction cups that provide a surprising amount of suction. These work quite well on nipples, and also on the clitoris if the submissive is female. Ordinary dental floss makes great nipple bondage. Tie a slipknot in a piece of dental floss and pull it snug on the submissive's nipples.

If you do decide to try dripping hot candle wax on your partner's naked body, make sure to use colourless paraffin wax candles the first few times you try it. Coloured candles have a higher melting point, and so the wax will hurt a lot more. Also be prepared for the fact that you will probably have to vacuum up afterwards, as the wax crumbles and gets everywhere once it dries. It is good fun but messy. Use a cheap vinyl tablecloth to cover the dining room table. Melt paraffin candles into a burner and brush the wax onto your lover's skin.

Remote-controlled vibrators and butt plugs are available at most sex toy stores these days. While they are fun to play with in their own right, in group or semi-public settings they are particularly effective. Submissives can be equipped with a remote-controlled toy, and then go out to dinner with friends. During the evening, the friends can take turns with the control, and the submissive can try to guess who has it.

Regular toys left in place for extended periods of time make it impossible for a slave to ignore the penetration, whatever else he or she may be doing. This in turn can keep the submissive constantly thinking about and constantly craving sexual stimulation. I have even made my lovers keep a dildo inserted as they sleep - which tends to make the night filled with non-stop erotic dreams. Of course, this can be adapted easily for male submissives as well, by having them sleep with a butt plug inserted.

Brushes of various sorts are excellent on bare skin, especially when the submissive is blindfolded. For example, a soft brush such as a shaving or make-up brush can be alternated with a stiff brush such as a toothbrush. Chinese writing brushes are an often overlooked but very effective toy. An electric toothbrush makes a wonderful sex toy when used on a clitoris. Try caressing your lover's skin with soft fur, coarse sandpaper, and other textures.

A bamboo barbecue skewer is an interesting sensation toy when used on a bound and blindfolded person. Dragged slowly and with moderate pressure over the skin, it feels much sharper than it is; used on sensitive areas like nipples and breasts, you can make someone believe that you are actually piercing the skin with a needle, even though the skewer is blunt and will not break skin.

Knives can make fun and psychologically powerful sex toys. You do not actually have to cut your partner in order to do knife play. A semi-sharp or pointed knife edge drawn over skin, not hard enough to break the skin, is an intense and erotically charged sensation - especially if it is combined with a blindfold. Draw the knife very slowly over your partner's body for an emotionally intense effect. A bit more intensity can be achieved by using a dull butter knife that has been kept in the freezer for a few hours. The cold edge makes it feel razor sharp. The back, chest, thighs, and legs are all excellent places for knife play.

Ice is a great all-purpose sex toy. Run an ice cube over your lover's body, especially if your lover is blindfolded and/or bound. Before penetrating anything with an ice cube, run water over it to prevent it from sticking to delicate membranes or place it in your mouth and run your lips and tongue over your lover's body. To make an ice dildo take a plain unlubricated condom and the cardboard tube from the centre of a roll of paper towels. Cut the cardboard tube lengthwise, then close it into a cylinder that is as wide as you want the dildo to be, and tape it. Fill the condom with water, tie it shut, and suspend it in the tube with a piece of string; the cardboard tube will prevent the water from bulging in the dildo. Then place it upright in the freezer for a few hours to create a seamless ice dildo. Bubble wrap is another way to make an unusual dildo. Take a length of bubble wrap and roll it tightly, bubble-side out for additional texture and place a condom over it with a rubber band or tape to hold it all in place in place.

There are many internet sites filled with ridiculously expensive hoods and masks but a simple gas mask from a military surplus store is often just as effective, thanks to its creepy psychological connotaions. Plague doctor masks made from papier-mâché can be just as intimidating if you are on a really tight budget.

In Fifty Shades of Grey, the heroes are rich, handsome, sexual dominants with a seemingly endless supply of money. They happily invest their fortunes in expensive contraptions, hidden pleasure rooms, and state-of-the-art sex toys to pleasure their female subs. Fortunately exploring BDSM and other sexual fantasies does not have to cost an arm and a leg (or any other interesting body part). DIY versions are often just as good as anything that is available in the expensive sex shops. The term "pervertable" refers to a common household item that can be "hidden in plain sight" and re-purposed for sex play with your partner. For example the common spatula delivers a powerful slap and leaves delicious fist-sized marks on your lover's backside. Try spray painting all of these items black so that they look the part. Seek out dollar stores, head-shops, weird craft stores, pet shops and haircare stores for all kinds of imaginative pervertables.

A plastic golf ball (the hollow type with airflow holes) and a piece of cord thread through the middle works just as well as any rubber ball gag. Alternative find a latex-coated foam ball, a pair of shoe laces, and a BBQ skewer. Heat the skewer over a gas stove or BBQ grill and steady the ball in a vice. Once the skewer is hot, begin inserting it into the ball, twisting as you go; reheat as needed until the skewer is all the way through and the hole is wide enough. Allow both the skewer and ball to cool completely. Then, use the skewer to force both shoelaces through and centre them through the ball. You now have a ball gag that can be tied both above and below the ears for extra security. Choking caused by the ball not being firmly attached to the part that buckles/ snaps/ties around a slave's head can otherwise be a real risk. This can be avoided by encasing the ball into a pair of tights/leggings and then tying the leggings around the back of the head.

One of my own most memorable sessions was with a translator named Aurora and a couple of fly swatters. The new slave was hog tied with her pert little derrière protruding rudely up into the air. I lifted up her blindfold for a moment so that she could see what I was going to beat her with. Her eyes almost popped out of their sockets when she saw the electric mosquito zapper, the thin wires stretched across its tennis racket style frame. I only had to touch it against the door handle and the crackling blue sparks had her screaming in terror. Thankfully the gag muffled her cries and prevented her from rousing the neighbours. I replaced her eye-shade and unbeknownst to her, switched to a standard plastic fly swatter. When it made contact with bare skin of her soft behind, I thought that she was going to hit the ceiling.

Pet stores carry lots of items that can be used in even more interesting ways if you have an imagination. I especially like the feathers attached to thin nylon rods in the cat toy section. The rods can be used as canes, while the feathers are great little sensuality devices. Pet stores have some very nice collars which are incredibly cheaper than anything you can find in a kink store. Remember, kink is a big profit business because they are catering to a specialized group and can therefore charge much higher prices.

Dice and cards can create an element of surprise and tension. Use index cards or blank business cards in conjunction with a punishment box. Each card has an erotic punishment written on it. If the submissive misbehaves, he or she has to draw a punishment card at random from the box. Have the submissive create the cards - preferably while aroused and they will think of all kinds devious things that would never otherwise occur to you. Review each one to make sure it is actually a punishment, and reject any that are really rewards in clever disguise. Make sure to punish the slave for each rejected card.

If you also have a reward box then add in a marble bag. Fill it with twenty marbles, ten black and ten white, but you can also use black and red checkers. If the slave draws a black marble, choose a card from the punishment box; if the slave chooses a white marble, choose a card from the reward box. This is very effective if, whenever the slave misbehaves, you take a white marble out of the bag and replace it with a black one. If they do anything exceptionally worthy of praise then add a white marble to the bag.

Talking dirty is fun; writing dirty things on your partner's body is even more fun. You can write something as simple as 'slut' across your partner's chest or you can write short descriptions of what you plan to do to your partner just before you do it. This can also be reversed; one person can write on his or her own body things he or she would like to have happen, and let his or her partner discover the writing as things progress. Write things like "property of so-and-so" in large letters on the chest, then send him or her to work that way.

Names are important. Female slaves usually address their owners by the title of "Master," indicating the difference of status between them. Surely no girl in bondage would dare use her master's name to address him. Such privilege is reserved for his peers. For the master 'Be silent, Slave!' is perfectly acceptable but a slave name is useful in adding realism to role-plays. In these fantasies, she is, commonly, someone else. Accordingly the name should be different. Furthermore, she must accept it. A slave has no say in the name which is given to her. It should be a name which makes her feel vulnerable and sexy; and a name which makes him feel sexually hot and aggressive. Sometimes an aristocratic name is good, the name contrasting with the lowliness of the slave who bears it.

Orgasm denial is a fun, and frustrating, technique that can bring some of the spark back into sex. Most women really enjoy getting guys very turned on and making them ask permission to cum, then saying no many times. Over time, the sexual tension builds up, and your partner becomes perpetually aroused. When done over a period of several days or longer, this technique creates a very powerful level of sexual excitement. When you do finally allow your partner release, it will be an extremely intense experience

Another exciting technique is to treat your partner like a living sex toy. Use him or her as a human sex doll and put them into different positions while they must remain completely passive, sometimes easier said than done. They are forbidden to make any sound or respond in any way whatsoever. Failure to remain completely passive earns a punishment.

One of the many books out there, I highly recommend Screw the Roses, Send Me The Thorns by Philip Miller and Molly Devon. This is a great overview of BDSM play, including introduction to basic safety tips, etc. For DIY freaks keen on making their own gear, 21st Century Kinkycrafts by Janet W. Hardy is available from the Greenery Press website or from Amazon.

Here are some more useful DIY gear links.

Fetlife.com is one of the most active DSDM forums of the internet

kinkacademy.com (unlike Fetlife, it is all professional educators)

Sartan's Working With Leather includes a list of tools, glues and materials and suppliers.

APPENDIX 3 - APPAREL IN SEXUAL FANTASIES

The female partner is usually the star of these erotic enactments and just as it is said that clothes make the man, they are equally effective in creating the most exciting sexual fantasies. Women can be endlessly inventive in these matters, and sometimes the details are best left to them. They can usually design costumes that are sensuous dreams.

Fortunately, there are now many items commercially available, which are, fantastically sexy. Consider, for example, the range of female nightwear: White classic garments which, when worn with a pair of barbaric armlets will transform her into a pagan warrior queen. Silky is always better than slutty and torrid always tops trashy. Torrid and trashy are two very different things.

Female underwear can often be adapted for certain scenarios, especially now that there is such a wide choice of styles available. The animal patterns of tiger and leopard skin are excellent when capturing a "Sheba of the Jungle," and turning her into a harem slave. These days it is possible to find zebra skin, Siberian tiger skin and even snow leopard prints. If you are kidnapping a Victorian lady aristocrat, and taking her to a rain forest hideaway as your personal sex-slave, you might want to give her garments fashioned from the skins of trophy animals that you yourself have hunted and killed. The fact that you bought them on the high street can be hidden by adding a little beading and fringing to them.

Swim wear is less appropriate, though a bikini that ties, and is easily removable, is good. A brief terry cloth cover-up, with absolutely nothing under it, is delightful. Generally, however, swim wear is less easy to remove. Diaphanous silk, half parted, brief and clinging beats even the most expensive bathing suit hands down. These are most commonly available in the form of nighties, of which there is a vast selection. With the short gowns, of course, the woman is not permitted to wear the panties. They are a cop-out, making the shortness of the gown meaningless.

Belly dancer outfits are widely available. It is for good reason that these wonderfully revealing costumes have been so popular for many hundreds if not thousands of years. The mysterious allure of a veil is unmistakable. The addition of a few extras such a head dress or finger cymbals makes them downright irresistible. Think about appropriate props too. An evil sheik would not look on from a futon or an Ikea sofa but lounge on silken cushions. He would probably be puffing on a hookah. Shisha water pipes are now quite easy to find and can add a great deal in accurately recreating a Bedouin encampment.

Rags can be wonderfully evocative; for example, the shreds of an old house dress, suitably ripped short and torn from the shoulder, etc., can be splendid. Such a rag, of course, must be her only garment. (Panties, incidentally, are never worn, unless they are all that is worn.)

"Of all these beautiful garments, Master, which will you give me to wear?" "None. You will wear the rags of a slave." An old slip or nightgown, suitably altered and shortened, can make an excellent slave garment. Consider a cord tied about her waist, in such a way that it can be casually yanked loose, supporting a rectangle of silk in the front and rear, thrust over and behind the cord. If it is desired a long piece of silk can be passed over the front cord, between her legs, and then up and under, and over, the cord in the back. It should then be made snug to her body. Separate pieces of silk are even sexier. These may be wider or narrower. They may be only a few inches in length, or they might reach below her knees, or even to her ankles. If there is only one such rectangle, perhaps it is a cultural norm in barbarian society that a slave girl's behind is always kept bared, perhaps the better to be switched in case of any misdemeanor. Alternatively a rectangle of cloth, with a hole cut out for the head, poncho fashion and thrown over the head makes a very effective slave garment. The sides are open. It can be belted with a rawhide thong. Its length is up to the players. My own feeling is the shorter the better.

Imagine a wench wearing only a narrow rectangle of red silk and a matching scarlet collar approaching you, to serve you wine. Women's breasts are beautiful, and they mark her so excitingly, vulnerably, as a female, it is a shame that our culture recommends their concealment. They are nothing to be ashamed of. I think we may suppose that, in many cultures supporting slavery, the slave girls would be forced, willing or not, to display their beauty for the pleasure of free men. Ankle bells, incidentally, can be sexy; the master knows where his wench is; she cannot surprise him; and, as she moves in love, the bells are exciting.

Costume changes in these fantasies can be stimulating. They also give the male a minute or two to cool off. Do not forget evening gowns, cocktail dresses, severe "business suits," etc. Women look lovely in them, and they are pleasures to remove, before putting her in, if anything, something more comfortable, more "suitable." An aristocratically dressed woman is a delight to strip. Perhaps the last things you remove are her pearls and earrings. Or perhaps you permit her to retain them, and then command her, still wearing them, to kneel before you. What about a scarlet halter, otherwise bare, save perhaps a matching strip of ribbon, tied about her left ankle? It should be, perhaps, two inches wide. (If she is nude, a man's wrist strap, with double buckles, fastened about her left ankle can be a lovely slave marking device. A small link chain, with padlock, can be another. A chain and padlock collar, too, is lovely.)

Do not forget leotards and body suits. They were clearly designed by someone interested in displaying the beauty of females. Leotards and body suits might, in many cultures, particularly those of the future, make excellent slave garments. Can you imagine the beauty, so clad, moving about among a clinically clean environment of highly complex computers? Full-body suits called zentai entirely immerse the wearer in skin tight fabric. The suits are essentially catsuits with gloves, feet, and a hood. The wearer experiences total enclosure and those who enjoy erotic objectification might make use of the garment's anonymizing aspect. The word zentai means whole body in Japanese. Japanese has a whole range of very useful sex related vocabulary. I like the Japanese term 'paizuri' for example because it sounds so much classier than 'tit-fucking'.

Garters are iconic sexual items and are inexpensive items that say just as much as any designer dress. Other budget priced accessories include gloves of any length, from a simple pair in white all the way up to full length black PVC, although these will obviously be considerably more expensive. You might be impressed at the impact of a matching pair of gloves, garters and high heels. Devastating would probably be a suitable description. Even the most simple items can be improved by adding a small red bow. This can range from a pair of bobby socks to a pair of white panties. Unfortunately the mark up on underwear and bedroom fashion is usually extortionate and so making your own is always a good way to save money. At the same time it allows you customise items to your very own stories and scenarios.

Brief, wrap-around skirts are excellent. What can be wrapped in one direction can be unwrapped in the other. Such garments can be removed in a very sexy fashion. They need not be climbed out of. The female can remove it gracefully, teasingly; humbly, obediently; in tears, in despair; insolently, whipping it from her, thrusting forward tauntingly; "I know I belong to you. I strip myself before you, your slave. You own me. Use me!" And so on.

It is important, too, not to neglect the hair. An obvious consideration here, applicable in some fantasies, is the transition from a severe, intellectual hair-do, appropriate to a man-hating blue stocking, to the wild, loose pelt of an untamed slave girl, perhaps on her hands and knees, stripped, looking up at you, in hatred, in fury, determined to resist. But she fears the whip in your hand. I personally like long, loose hair in a slave girl, exciting, uninhibited, sexy, wild, barbaric, uncivilized. I also like the feel of it on my body. Doubtless an aware slave girl uses her hair to please and stimulate her master.

Perhaps a house slave must braid her hair in a certain way, whereas a sex slave must wear her hair in a different fashion. Hair can be used, too, for signals. Perhaps when a slave girl wears her hair in a certain fashion, or, say, wears a certain pin in it, that is a wordless signal that she is begging for attention. The "bondage knot" might be of interest here, used in some slave cultures. Some strands of her hair, say, about a half inch, or an inch's worth, are separated from the rest and, loosely, knotted. The knot falls at her right cheekbone. This can be used as a general mark that the female is a slave, say, in lieu of collar, or as a special mark that she, fearing to speak, desires to be used as what she is, her master's girl. The master also, of course, could approach her, and tie this knot in her hair, she then understanding that she is to prepare herself.

Do not forget perfumes and lipsticks. Both are sexually stimulating. Lipstick, of course, in the sweet games, can be smeared, and mark pillows, etc. Perfume does not smear. Perhaps, by agreement among the players, certain perfumes and shades of lipstick have certain significances. Is a certain perfume, for example, slave perfume? Similarly, different characters might have different tastes. I once took a girlfriend away for the weekend and she brought body paint and cinnamon heat activated oil. It could have been been a wonderfully romantic weekend, but we wound up looking like Indians on the warpath with bulls-eye nipples and greasy burning genitalia.

There has been an explosion in sex shops and bondage boutiques. When I was young, rubber, leather and PVC outfits were only available in very specialist shops on Camden High Street or from obscure mail order catalogues. These days if it is not available on the high street, it can certainly be found on eBay or any number of fetish websites. The only problem is that a lot of this gear is still ridiculously expensive. I like PVC catsuits as much as the next man but sadly I am not one of these playboy millionaires that can drop a thousand dollars on a custom outfit which will only see a handful of outings. Instead I prefer to be more selective with my purchases a look for financial value over sheer shock value. Vintage clothes stores are my first choice for all kinds of unusual role playing outfits. Thrift stores and charity shops occasionally have interesting items but keeping an active eye on eBay is probably a more effective strategy.

The current cosplay explosion is making more fantasy outfits available than ever before. Suddenly quality costumes that were previously only found in movie studios are now for sale to ordinary consumers. As demand and manufacturing technologies continue to improve prices will inevitably drop even further. As well as cosplay, the LARP (Live Action Role Playing) community is a fantastic source of historical and fantasy costumes. From steam-punk explorers to medieval princesses, there are many periods and genres to choose from.

At one time, I was lucky enough to have a geeky girlfriend who loved science fiction, horror, and superhero comics. I had a black nylon cape and a white lab coat. She, in black lingerie and black cape, would be the super heroine who had been captured by the mad scientist. I would tie her up and play with her, coaxing out her true inner desires. Her "struggle" and eventual surrender were delicious. The next time around we reversed roles and she played the captor, immobilising the superhero and lavishing me with with her evil attentions. A superhero outfit combined with a Mexican wrestling mask and huge rubber gloves is bizarre and disturbing and erotic all at the same time. I urge you to give this strange combination a try and I think that you will be very pleasantly surprised. On the occasion that I came home from a cosplay convention dressed as Alex from A Clockwork Orange, my partner at the time enjoyed the most fulfilling rape fantasy of her entire life.

In the 1970s, the uniform's association with sadomasochism and forbidden sexuality was embodied in a wave of violent Nazisploitation films such as Ilsa, She-Wolf of the SS and the controversial art-house film The Night Porter (1974). In the latter film, a topless Charlotte Rampling has an iconic scene performing a Marlene Dietrich song for a group of concentration camp guards while wearing parts of an SS uniform. Her ensemble of army boots and pants, suspenders, peaked cap, and black opera gloves has been imitated countless times, most notably in pop singer Madonna's banned "Justify My Love" video in 1990. Boots of all kinds are even more sexy in bed that they are outside. Spurs if you can find them, make a very distinctive sound when walking and have an extremely arousing effect on many people.

Oriental outfits have a very seductive charm all of their own. Kimonos with their complex obis and extensive make-up are perhaps a little too troublesome for casual users yet Chinese qipaos and cheongsams are simple but effective. The combination of high collar and short skirt is delicious and can be complimented with lots of overdone eye make-up and a pair of chopsticks to tie up the hair. An simple silk 'ao dai' and a conical bamboo hat can be effective if you want to recreate some kind of Vietnam scenario. I am sure that you can find plenty of Hollywood inspiration from Full Metal Jacket and Apocalypse Now. A lesser know item of Chinese female costume is the duduo. Literally translated as a stomach cover, this handkerchief-size garment is a type of ancient Chinese underwear, a bra alternative first worn in the Ming and Qing Dynasties. Unlike bras today, the dudou was worn to flatten the breasts as flat-chested women were thought to be graceful while busty women were considered a temptation. A dudou resembles a small square or diamond shaped apron. They are backless and have strings that tie around the neck and back and are made of brightly coloured silk or crepe and are sometimes embellished with embroidered flowers and butterflies. Designs of tigers, scorpions, snakes and geckos were embroidered to ward off evil spirits. Themes of love, such as lotus and pairs of mandarin ducks, were also common. Some dudou have a pocket in which to keep ginger, musk or other Chinese medicinal herbs believed to keep the belly warm. International fashion designers including Versace and Miu Miu have created their own versions, with Versus designing a dudou of pink leather. Very small tops such as dudous need to be worn with long trousers or a long skirt to look elegant and achieve some balance.

As a man, I like to dress up just as much as my partner. I have always been fascinated by fancy dress parties and relish to opportunity to take on the role of a character that is so much larger than life. I especially enjoy challenging convention and wearing items that are beyond the usual norms. Some of these, such as the kilt, work very well in bedroom fantasies. When you are role-playing a marauding Mel Gibson as Braveheart or a bloodstained, triumphant gladiator it is important to remember that trousers were a comparatively recent invention. For many millennia, even the most macho men wore skirts, long before pants came on to the scene. It is only in the last few hundred years that they have dropped out of fashion but even now you will find celebrities and cutting-edge sub-genres reinventing the male skirt. Punks and cybergoths flaunt their androgyny with everything from small bum flaps to vast leather bondage skirts complete with studs, straps and zippers. Two of the most exciting kilt manufacturers on the market at the moment are Utilikilts and Kiltthis. Both companies produces a range of ultra-macho leather kilts that look amazing with a pair of work boots and a bike jacket. They are admittedly quite expensive but there are kilt patterns all over the internet and they are surprisingly easy to make for yourself. I especially like the DPM camouflage designs or the black leather that looks like something out of Game of Thrones.

Perhaps even more specialist but still my favourite are Tibetan clothing styles. I am not talking here about the saffron robes of the Dalai Lama but the bright colours and thick furs of Khampa cowboys and Himalayan swordsmen. Warriors of the plateau are often seen stripped to the waist with their chuba jackets tied around their hips as skirts. Tibetans are legally permitted to carry knives and it is still common to see burly nomads armed with huge swords in Shangri La or Gyantse. It might just be my personal preference but Tibetan Princesses wear a regalia that makes other royal costumes pale in comparison. Fabulously embroidered silks, thick mountain furs and many kilos of semi-precious stones make for some of the most brightly coloured outfits that you will ever see. Perhaps not for everybody but this is my book so I might as well include my own personal favourite outfits while I have the chance.

APPENDIX 4 -
ENVIRONMENTS AND
INSPIRATIONS

Candlelight gives a warm, loving glow, soft and intimate. Do not hesitate to make love by candlelight. The light from an open hearth is also very beautiful, of course, and barbaric. It can suggest a cave fire or the blaze in the hall of a Viking chieftain, especially with a thickly piled, heavy animal rug before the fire, on which to lie. On this rug, the captured thrall, naked save for a collar and chains looks magnificent. Torchlight, is sexy and atmospheric. Unfortunately most modern houses and apartments do not come equipped with wall cressets or other types of torch mountings. These days we seem to prefer electric light bulbs. The main problem with torches is that they have a tendency to blacken the ceiling with smoke, if not burn down the entire house, something that could be extremely inconvenient and embarrassing to explain to an insurance company. Some Halloween costume shops sell black bowls with mini fans inside that blow up a piece of orange silk. These give the impression of a flaming cauldron and can be used as a perfectly good substitute if you a trying to recreate the cave of a sabre-tooth tiger or a medieval oubliette. If your fantasy is set in the Victorian or Edwardian period, then gas lamps are relatively easy to find. Fanny by gaslight is indeed an intoxicating sight

Deep down, almost every man fancies himself a ruler who will subjugate women. The Chinese and Mongols had courts where the emperor had his pick of hundreds or thousands of concubines. Men were outright murdered or made eunuchs to serve in the emperor's court, and many more were sent off to fight in the many petty wars between warring factions. In the medieval age, the European feudal lords had sex with your wife before you did, right after the wedding.

He controlled your entire life and he would probably go on to have sex with your daughters. Some of the Ottoman sultans had large harems where they had their pick of many, many women. In South American pre-European empires leaders of men were given a proportion of women close to how many men they led. Meaning the bigger the tribe you led, the more women of that tribe you got to have sex with. Think Bathsheba of the Bible, Helen of Troy, Cleopatra of Egypt, any knight in shining armour rescues princess variant (Mario games, medieval stories, bed time stories, etc.), any action movie where the guy kills hundreds of guys and endures torture just to have sex with the girl in the end, and so on. The list is never ending.

The rrotic fantasy sub-genre, as the name suggests, contains strong sexual elements. Erotic fantasy is not so much defined by its story as by its scenes—which include numerous and much more graphic sex scenes. There are some "erotic" fantasies which are thinly veiled porn novels, while others maintain the importance of elements like plot, characters, and story. Here are a few to introduce you to the genre

Kushiel's Dart by Jacqueline Carey.
The first novel in a six-part series, this is an epic tale that features a female protagonist who is both spy and courtesan. She has been chosen to experience pain and pleasure as one.

Centuries Ago and Very Fast by Rebecca Ore.
A series of stories that are linked by a time jumping, gay immortal. The stories span centuries and feature many lovers.

The Iron Dragon's Daughter by Michael Swanwick.
A young girl escapes a factory that makes iron dragons and embarks on a journey of rebellion. The protagonist is a strong female character, she is angry and she tries to enjoy herself in a dark world (i.e. sex).

Palimpsest by Catherynne Valente.
Palimpsest is a rich and intoxicating world that only a select few

are able to reach. It is a dreamy world and the map is attained by having an orgasmic experience.

The Unlimited Dream Company by J.G. Ballard.
A surreal story about death and transformation, about freedom and escape, and quite a bit of mating. Told by an unreliable narrator who just may be insane and who becomes a kind of pagan-like god.

The Sleeping Beauty by A.N. Roquelaure.
A trilogy actually written by Anne Rice using a pen name that very loosely follows the Sleeping Beauty fairy tale. It takes places in a medieval fantasy world and explicitly describes the sexual adventures of Beauty as well as other male characters.

Bound by Sophie Oak.
The first novel in this series begins with an ordinary woman being kidnapped and taken to a magical and fantastical world to be bonded with twin brothers who share a soul.

The Gor Series by John Norman. About a third of the way through the series, the publisher changed from Del Rey to Daw Books, Inc. With the release of Hunters of Gor, book number eight, the slavery aspect became much more prominent. The covers had always been erotic S/M fantasy themes but now the books were filled with that kind of imagery too. In turn, Norman found Planet of the Apes, based on the book by Pierre Bouille particularly compelling. In this work, apes are the dominant species and hunt the primitive humans, keeping them as slaves. "The Bouille fantasy incorporates a number of elements indicative of the successful fantasy. It is detailed, and deliberate. It is carefully worked out. It gains a reality in virtue of the very multiplicity and obduracy of the detail which defines it. It is a congruent, appropriate, natural series of events in a congruent, appropriate, natural environment. It is a bizarre real happening in a bizarre real world. Furthermore, it incorporates hazard, capture, helplessness and forced sex."

In the digital age, remember that a well chosen soundtrack can always add so much more to a fantasy scenario. Take advantage of music sharing software such as Soulseek to locate music and special effects that are relevant and pertinent to the fantasy that you are re-enacting. Think of Gregorian chant for medieval setting or the ethereal sounds of Phaedra by Tangerine Dream for a futuristic punishment cube.

About the Author

Darby Jones first began writing as a teenager, when he quickly displayed an early talent for penning sensuous erotica and hard-core porn. For many years he was a prolific contributor to UK magazines such as Mayfair, Fiesta and Knave, as well as a host of lesser known but equally popular titles. After a short stint at Viz Comics, he left England to become the lead contributor of an infamous but long out-of-print travel opus, entitled Sex Havens for Tax Fiends. This was a strictly limited edition, leather-bound gazetteer commissioned by the now defunct Scope Publications. It was published as a follow up to their extremely popular PT (Perpetual Traveller) titles, including as The Passport Report, The Honorary Consul and The Invisible Investor. Each volume immediately sold out and remains highly collectible to this day.

For the last three years, he has been enjoying forced early-retirement after an extremely stressful eighteen months smuggling Chinese-made arms and munitions to the various rebel groups in Eastern and Northern Myanmar. He was forced to spend nearly a year in Malaysia recuperating from a near-fatal gun-shot injury, which was sustained in a shoot-out on the upper reaches of the Mekong. He is currently in an undisclosed Asian location working on his latest book.